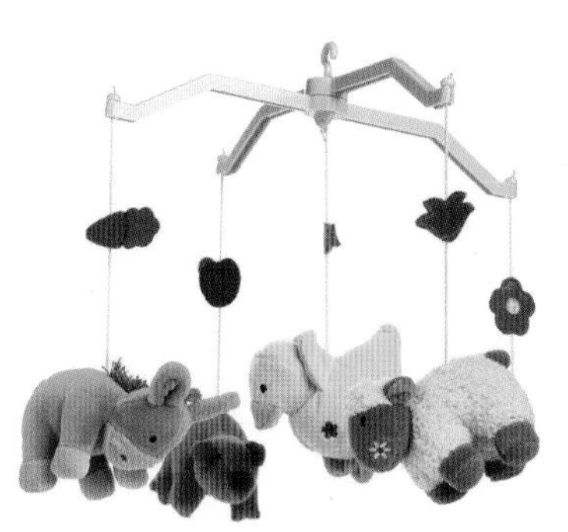

Help your baby to sleep

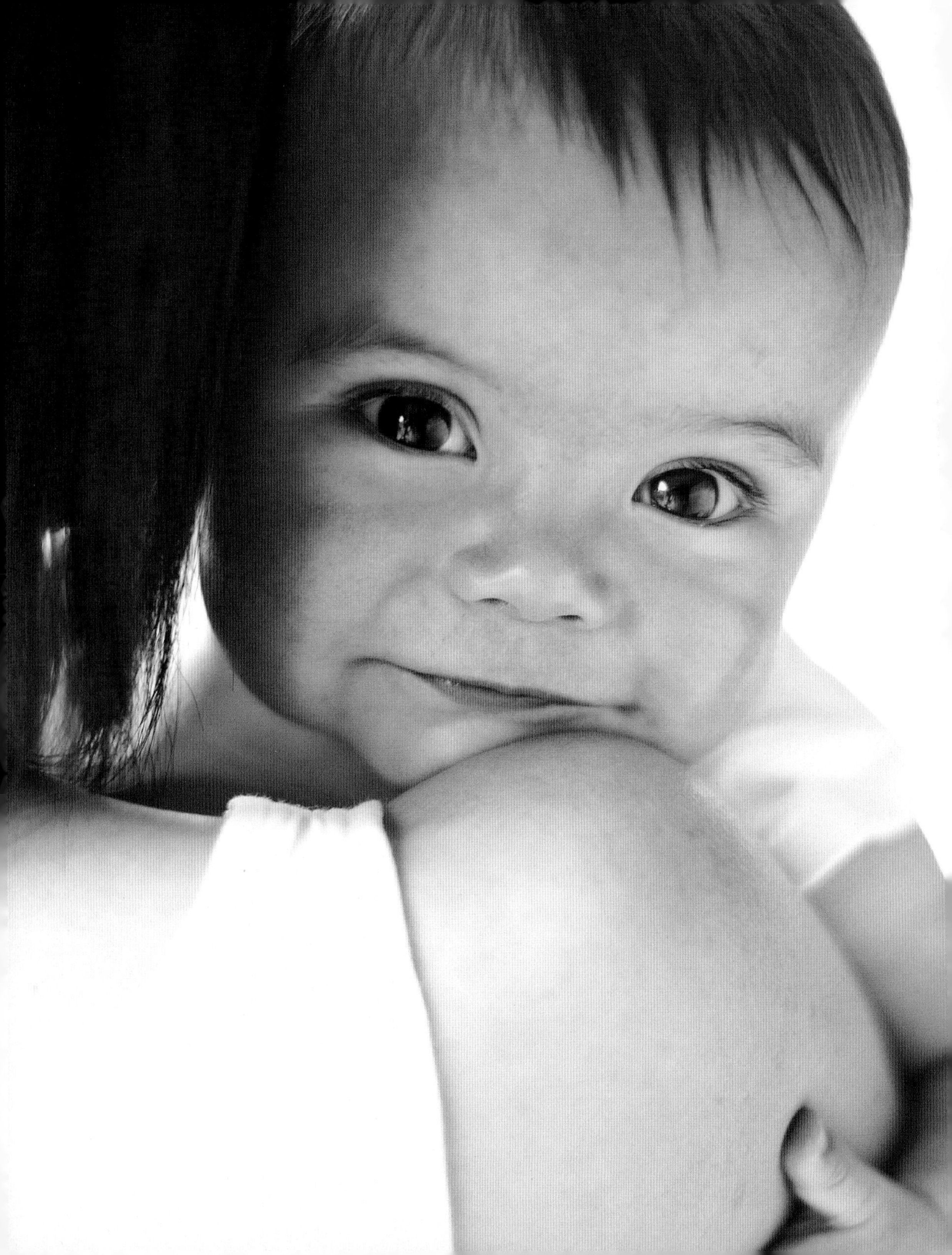

Help your baby to sleep

Practical sleep solutions, from newborn to age three

Judy Barratt

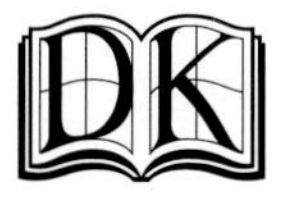

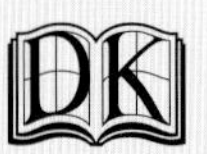

LONDON, NEW YORK,
MELBOURNE, MUNICH, AND DELHI

Project editor Claire Cross
Art editor Vanessa Hamilton
Illustrator Vanessa Hamilton
Jacket designer Saskia Janssen
Pre-production producer Andy Hilliard
Senior producer Jen Scothern
Creative publishing manager Anna Davidson
Creative director Jane Bull
Publisher Peggy Vance
Special sales creative project manager
Alison Donovan

Every effort has been made to ensure that the information in this book is complete and accurate. However, neither the publisher nor the authors are engaged in rendering professional advice or services to the individual reader. The contents of this book are not intended as a substitute for consulting with your healthcare provider. All matters regarding the health of you and your child require medical supervision. Neither the publisher nor the authors shall be liable or responsible for any loss or damage allegedly arising from any information or suggestions in this book.

First published in Great Britain in 2014
by Dorling Kindersley Limited
80 Strand, London WC2R 0RL

A Penguin Random House Company

2 4 6 8 10 9 7 5 3 1

001 – 270955 – Sept/14

A CIP catalogue record for this book
is available from the British Library.

ISBN 978-0-2410-1084-6

Printed and bound in China by
Leo Paper Products Ltd.

Discover more at
www.dk.com

Contents

Introduction

Each of us has unique sleep patterns, needs, and preferences – a newborn has different sleep needs to a toddler, who has different needs to you. For family life to function efficiently, lovingly, and healthily, you need to align everyone's sleep as much as you can. With a new baby that begins with teaching her that daytime is for wakefulness, and the nighttime for sleep.

A recent study in West Virginia, USA, revealed that most new mothers are awake for around two hours every night feeding or comforting a new baby. How can you get back that sleep debt? And how can you teach your baby good sleep habits to minimize the period of her life when she wakes in the night? Those are just the beginnings of the myriad sleep-related questions most parents will have over the course of their baby's childhood. What happens when your baby gets a bit older and doesn't want to go to sleep when you say? What effects will a growing imagination have on her – and your – sleep? How can you set her up with a lifetime of good sleep habits that mean not just better health for her now and in the future, but for all of you, because you will all benefit from her improved sleep? And what strategies can you put in place to try to turn a poor sleeper into a child who sleeps like the proverbial baby? The questions go on.

This book begins with an overview of sleep and why it is important. Chapter One encourages you to think about what you and your partner (and any other children) need from sleep, and to consider the goals for your baby's sleep. We also look at many of the common concerns parents have about teaching their baby to sleep, as well as thinking about ways to repay your own sleep debt.

Then, chapter by chapter, the book takes you from newborn to toddlerhood, explaining the changes in your baby's sleep cycles and needs as she grows. For each age-group, it looks at all aspects of "sleep hygiene" – the fundamental principles we need to follow to gain a good night's sleep, which you can put in place for your baby from her earliest days. Among them are the sleeping environment (your baby's bed; her room; noise levels; and the effects of light and darkness) and the little rituals that prepare your baby for sleep. Each chapter also looks at age-specific sleep stealers, such as growth spurts, bedtime resistance, nighttime wakefulness, and nightmares and night terrors.

Learning to sleep well starts in the first few weeks of life.

In Chapter Seven, we look at the major sleep-training methods, providing an instant reference so that you can assess sleep problems, find the most appropriate technique for overcoming them, and implement them with the knowledge of what to expect and how long you might have to wait for an outcome. No one method works for every baby and every family in every situation. As sleep itself is unique to each of us, so are the solutions to sleep problems. Throughout the book the aim is to help you make informed decisions about how best to implement strategies and techniques for sleeping success for your baby, and for you, too.

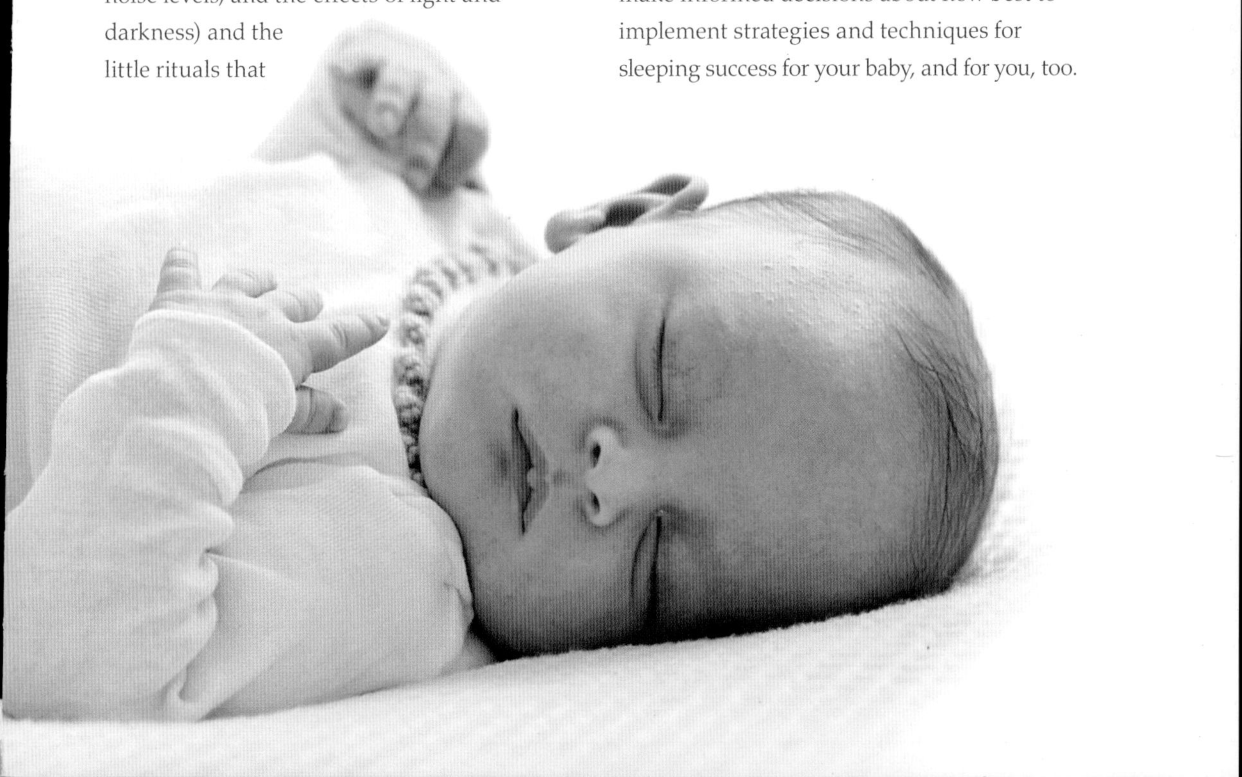

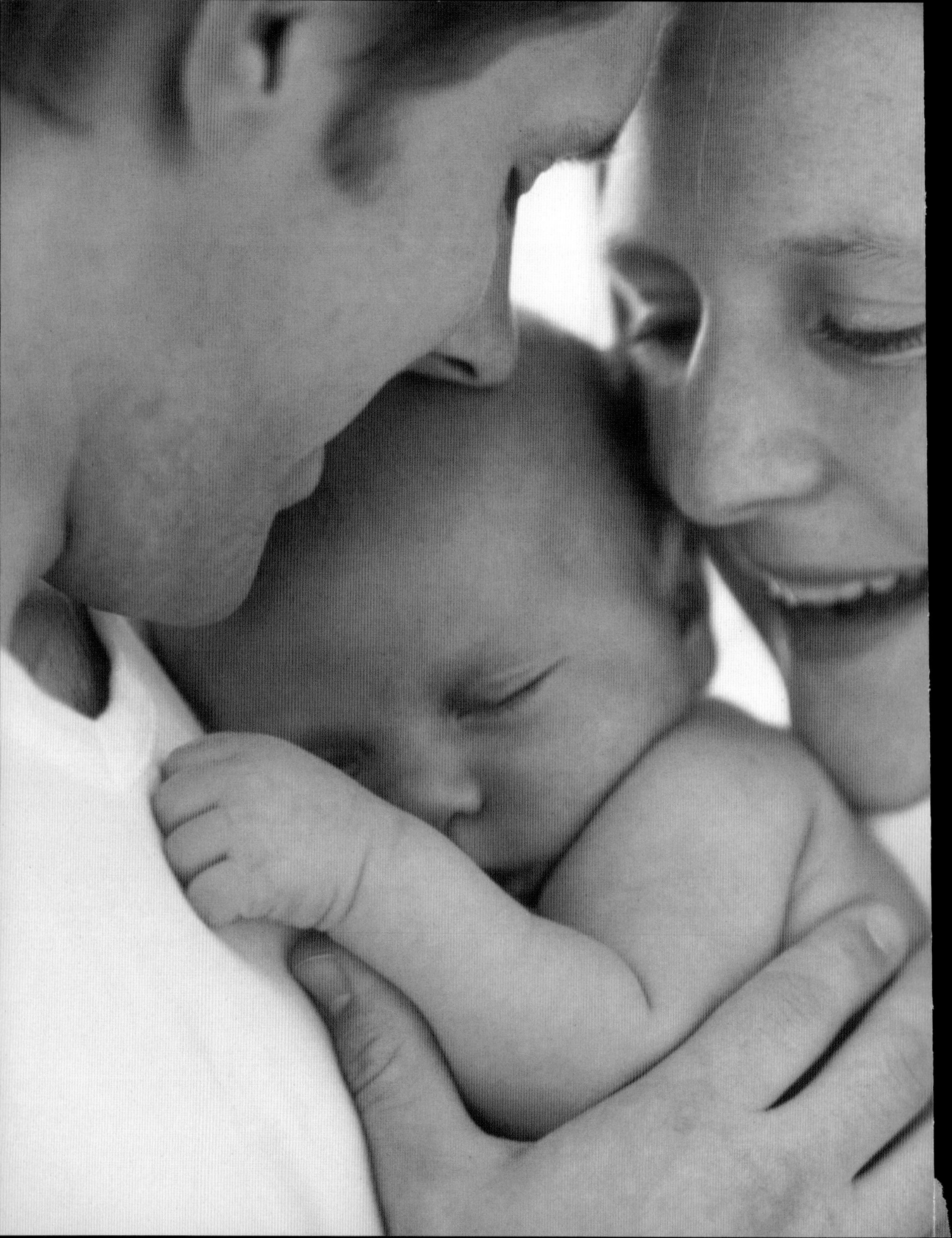

1

Sleep and your family

It's a cliché, but nothing prepares you for the upheaval of life with a new baby. This tiny being, probably not much longer than your lower arm, impacts everything from when you eat to when you leave the house – to when you sleep. Before you look into methods for teaching your baby to sleep in a way that suits both of you, it's essential to understand two things: first, why sleep is important for you and for your baby; and, second, what variables you will need to decide upon in order to take a consistent approach to getting the best sleep patterns from your baby – for your health, your baby's health, and the health and lifestyle of your whole family.

Why sleep is important

If you have a newborn, or an older baby or toddler who isn't yet sleeping through the night, you'll be only too aware of the effects of sleep deprivation on yourself, and on your child, too. While it's possible for the body to rest during waking hours, sleep is a vital component of our lives for a whole variety of reasons.

Why we sleep

We all need sleep to function at optimal levels during the day. You have probably seen innumerable government warnings about the dangers of driving when you're tired. Sleep enables you to clear your mind for the start of the new day, improving alertness, productivity, and creativity. If you are looking after a baby, you need your sleep so that you can be attentive, responsible, at your best, and able to fulfil his needs. For your baby, sleep improves his waking alertness for all the learning that he has to do, and, as he develops, makes sure that his coordination is in tip-top condition so that he is less likely to hurt himself, for example by tripping over. Studies show that children who get less than 10 hours sleep a night tend to have an increased risk of daytime injury.

Sleep provides an essential time for consolidation. When we sleep, the brain gathers together the day's learning, then creates memories and stores knowledge that might be useful in the future. This applies as

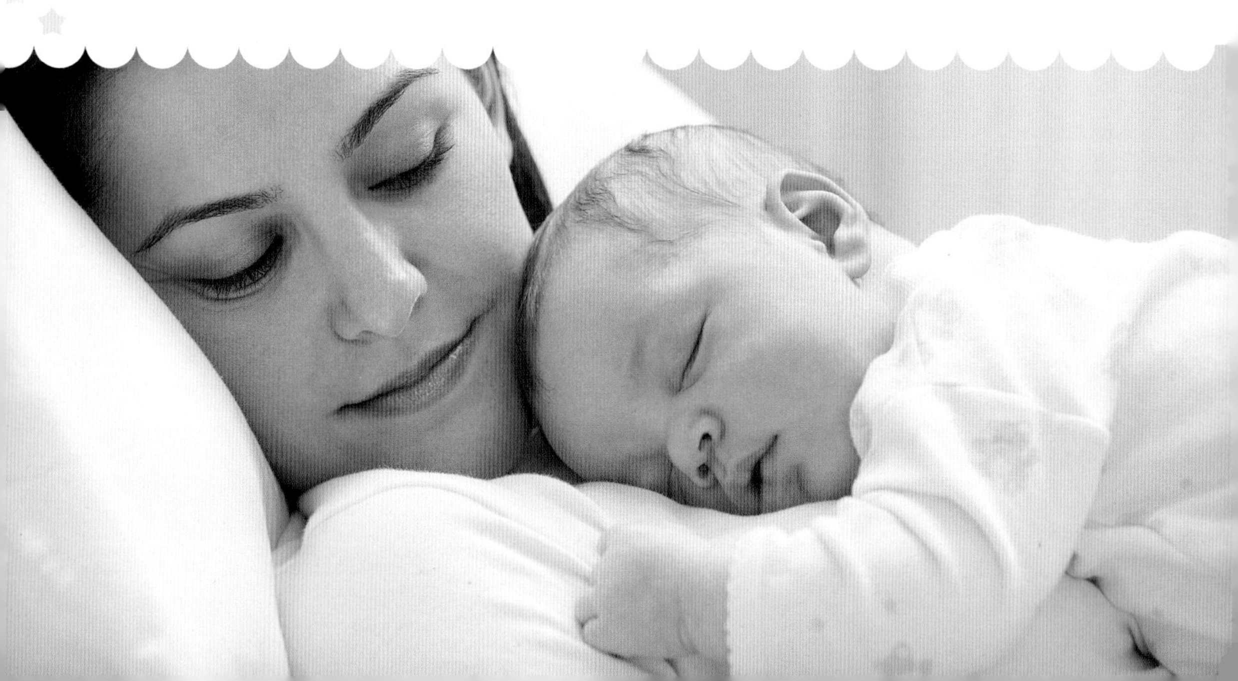

Understanding sleep

Every living thing sleeps, even plants. For hundreds of years, scientists and philosophers have been trying to work out why exactly we need sleep. The answer is that sleep is vital for growth, regeneration, and consolidation.

much to anything you might learn at work or from reading a book, as it does to the information your baby gathers simply by being awake and looking around, absorbing all the new sights, smells, tastes, and feelings that being in the world has to offer.

The third most important function of sleep is to give the body time to undertake essential physical repair or regeneration without distraction. Whether you are suffering from the early stages of a cold or have torn a muscle or ligament, or if you are a baby and need to grow and develop, as you sleep, energy that might during waking hours keep you on the move is diverted to fighting disease, repairing injury, and enabling growth.

Your sleep, your baby's sleep

Young or old, as darkness falls (this is important), your pineal gland, which lies in the lower part of your brain, releases the hormone melatonin. This sets your biological clock and signals to your body that nighttime is coming and it's time to sleep. Your brain receives and understands the message and sets off a sequence of events in your body that induce sleep. At the same time, your body temperature begins to fall, and it is while it is dropping most rapidly that you fall asleep.

It's at this point – the moments between waking and sleeping – that your sleep and your baby's sleep begin to follow different patterns. If you are a healthy sleeper, you will have a single, long period of sleep characterized by four or five "sleep cycles", each one roughly 90 minutes in length. Each of your sleep cycles takes you through drowsy, to light, to deep, to dreaming sleep, and

Your young baby needs to feed regularly throughout the night in the first few months.

between each cycle you will have a brief awakening, which you probably won't even notice. Babies have much shorter sleep cycles, of only 45 minutes to an hour, made up of only deep or dreaming sleep (this changes as your baby gets older). Like you, your baby will wake briefly between each cycle – but he is less able to drop back off without noticing he woke up. In parents, certain bodily functions shut down during sleep, including, in general, the need to go to the loo and the need to eat. For babies, though, toileting and feeding are still very much primal instincts, and nothing as mundane as sleep – their own or a parent's – is going to stand in the way of either.

Thinking about your sleep

Studies show that, while there is some genetic predisposition as to whether or not a baby becomes a good sleeper or a restless sleeper, getting your baby to sleep through the night is largely down to teaching. As with most matters related to children, consistency is key, so it's worth spending time, ideally before the birth, thinking about what sleeping set-up works for you, your family, and your lifestyle.

Your own sleeping patterns

Are you a lark or an owl? Can you function efficiently on six or seven hours sleep a night, or are you someone who needs a full nine hours? Are you happy to nap during the day when your baby naps? What about your partner's sleep patterns? What time do you each need to get up in the morning? And if you're a single parent, will you need to adapt your sleep patterns to work with your baby's?

Often the first barrier to helping your baby to sleep is getting everyone's objectives aligned. Think about your sleep needs and those of your partner so that together you can manage to work with your baby's own sleep patterns.

Once you've established what you both need from your sleep, work out the best sleeping place for your baby, and (if you aren't breastfeeding) a way to share the nighttime load. Decide, too, what parameters you will set in terms of soothing at night (what level of interaction with your baby feels comfortable, and who will do the soothing), with the aim of getting your baby to self-soothe as quickly as possible. Also discuss practical matters such as whether your baby should have a nightlight.

Working out your joint needs will help you and your partner to find a sleep arrangement to suit you all.

Who sleeps where?

Expert guidelines recommend that your baby sleeps in the same room as you until he is six months old to reduce the risks of Sudden Infant Death Syndrome, or SIDS (see p23).

If you are keeping your baby in your room with you, consider where in the room he will sleep. Here are some options:

- In a cot with a dropdown side that you can position up against your bed. This makes it easy to pull your baby close for breastfeeding, but you must be certain that there are no gaps that your baby could fall into between the cot and the bed.
- In a Moses basket, crib, or cot beside your bed, which means you have to reach over to soothe your baby, or bring him in to your bed to feed.
- In a Moses basket, crib, or cot, but in another part of the room, away from your bed, which would mean you would have to get out of bed

to feed or soothe, but will reduce the likelihood that you will be disturbed by your baby's quietest snuffles and any fidgeting at night. Also your breathing and turning, and the smell of your breast milk, are less likely to disturb him.

- In your bed with you (which can be convenient if you are breastfeeding).

If you decide to have your baby in your bed, will your partner sleep there, too? Or will you agree that on week nights, for example, you sleep separately, if possible, so that one of you can get an uninterrupted night in another room? Perhaps (if you're not breastfeeding at night), you'll alternate who sleeps next to or in the room with your baby, so that neither of you goes a whole week without a full night's sleep. Or perhaps you'll swap at weekends only: if one of you is working during the week, that parent can give the co-sleeper a break.

On the other hand, the notion of sleeping separately from your partner may seem unnatural, unsupportive or unloving to both of you – you're in this together, after all. In which case, think of ways to support each other's, and your baby's, needs while you all sleep in one room. The positioning of the cot, where you feed at night – in bed or in a chair? – and whether or not you co-sleep are all important points to discuss and agree on.

With or without a light?

Another important decision to make is whether or not you will use a nightlight. The transition from light to dark is essential for setting your baby's body clock (see pp26–7). However, there are practical reasons why having a nightlight is a good idea – if you're

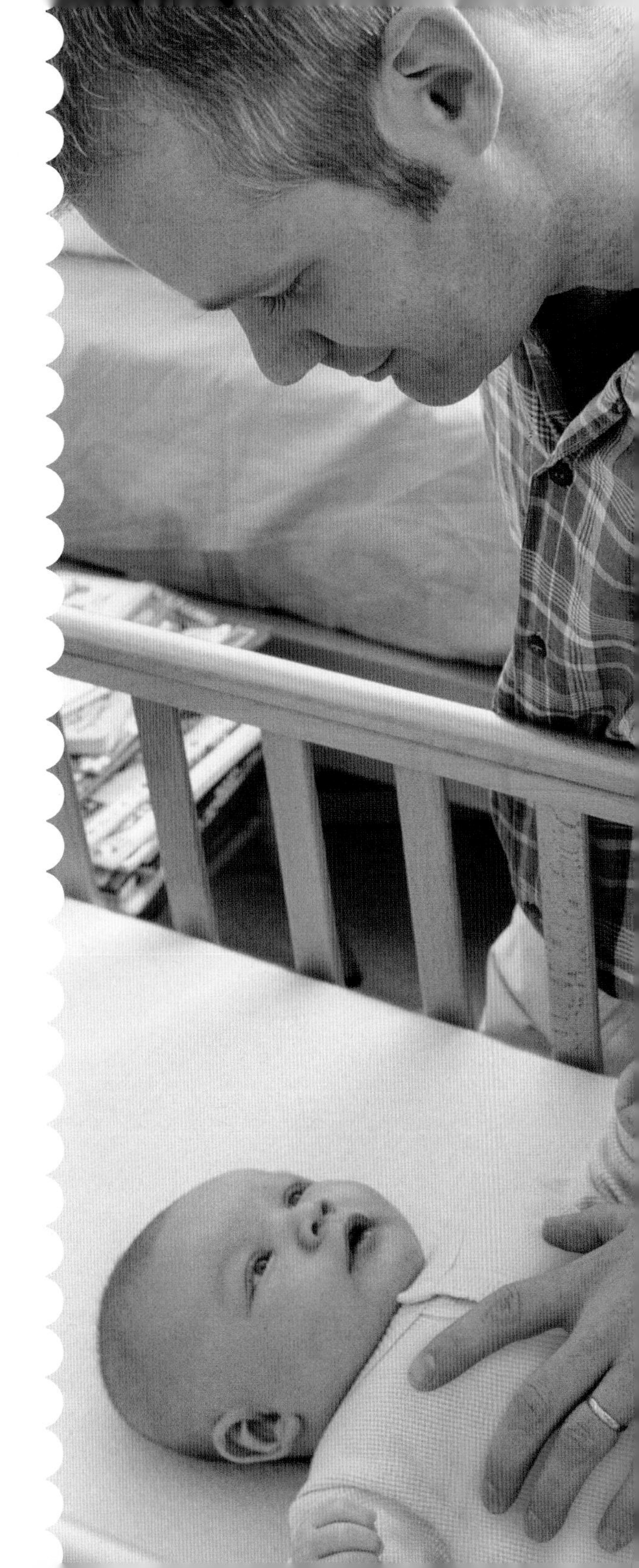

Essential learning

Studies show that long-term sleep problems can lead to poor concentration, obesity, and even aggression. Helping your baby to adopt healthy sleep habits is an important part of keeping him healthy for life.

bottle-feeding at night, you may need to see the bottle warmer or be able to establish how much of a feed your baby has had. Perhaps you need low-level light to reassure yourself that your baby is sleeping safely, and not tangled in his blanket. It's perfectly normal for older babies and toddlers to get a little bit unnerved at being plunged into darkness – perhaps a nightlight will ease the transition to their own room. Again, talk it through, make a plan, and then stick to it.

Your older child may wake for comfort and reassurance.

Comfort and reassurance

Babies cry when they are hungry, tired, or wet, but also when they are lonely. In the early weeks, your baby is most likely to need a feed when he wakes in the night as his tiny tummy can hold only a small amount of food, so he needs to feed every two to three hours around the clock. As he grows, he may wake increasingly for comfort. If you do not want to co-sleep, or you've decided to put your baby into another room to sleep, establish how you will go about soothing him when he wakes for no reason other than reassurance that someone else is there. Will you go into the room and pick him up for a cuddle, or will you offer a gentle pat or a stroke to indicate your presence? Whatever you decide, make sure that anyone who might be called upon to soothe your baby at night follows the same pattern of reassurance, with the ultimate aim that your baby will, in time, learn to soothe himself back to sleep.

Older babies and toddlers

If you have been through those early months, and are trying to help your older baby or your toddler to sleep better, it's more important than ever that you and your partner sit down to discuss what you both need and how you think you can best manage. Harness your need for sleep and use this as a motivation to find a system that you are both happy with, and which you think will be right for your baby. You may decide to avoid physical contact, instead offering a calming "shhh" – in which case, will you do this inside the room, or from the doorway? Whichever you prefer, make a plan (Chapter Seven can help you decide which settling approach might work for you) and then resolve to stick to it. With a newborn, you are forming good sleeping habits from the start, but with older babies and toddlers, you're trying to undo habits that may be established. An older baby who can't settle may be labelled "alert" and not in need of much sleep. In fact, overtired babies can be hyperactive. Spotting these signs can help you to unpick problem patterns and find long-term solutions. Sleep is both natural and essential for all of you, and as long as you go about teaching your child to sleep in a loving, reassuring manner, you will be improving not only your own wellbeing, but also that of your entire family.

When planning sleeping arrangements, try to look ahead to how things may change and adapt.

Consider the future

Whatever decisions you make about the family sleeping arrangements, try to look beyond the present and imagine what things will be like months from now. If you're certain you want to co-sleep (see pp22–3), think about when you may want this to stop, and how you will deal with moving your baby into his own sleeping space. Similarly, do you always want your child to have a nightlight, or would you like to phase this out in case he develops a fear of the dark? And are you prepared to pick up your baby to soothe him to sleep whenever he wakes? Even healthy sleepers may wake in the night well into their first decade of life, and although that seems a lifetime away when cradling your newborn, the more prepared you are for the changes ahead, the more likely you are to begin on a healthy and sustainable path.

Keeping a sleep diary

There are two good reasons to keep a sleep diary. First, it makes a good place to write down the key decisions that you and your partner make about how to tackle sleep in your family. Helping your baby to settle is, at times, hard work. A written note of the plans you had made is something to turn to when your resolve slips, or you're too tired to remember what you agreed. Second, keeping a note of the hours your baby sleeps – and, importantly, when – can help to map out the natural pattern of your baby's sleep. Working with that rhythm, even if you slowly try to shift it – minutes at a time – to better suit your own, can help to make the process of aligning your sleep patterns altogether easier.

Common concerns

Although some babies are naturally good sleepers, most have at least one period during which sleep is erratic or unpredictable. Lack of sleep, coupled with the inevitable insecurities of being a parent, can mean that at times it's hard to believe you're following the right path. Here, we look at some of the most common concerns parents have about their babies' sleep.

When should I start a bedtime routine?

Experts agree that there is very little you can do to teach your baby to sleep in any particular pattern in the first few weeks of life. Instead, follow your baby's lead and sleep when he sleeps. In the early days and weeks, you can start to introduce the notion of day and night (see pp26–7) and, at around six weeks, introduce a bedtime routine. Even though your baby may appear not to respond to these nighttime triggers yet, stick with them because, eventually, at somewhere around two or three months old, your consistency should start to pay off.

Should I leave my baby to cry?

A newborn baby has instinctive needs – for sustenance, love, and, of course, sleep. In the first few weeks and months after birth, your baby doesn't try to "manipulate" you – he merely tries to communicate his needs to you in the only way he knows how. It's important to respond, because in doing so you will help your newborn to feel secure in you and his new world. With a sense of security comes the confidence to know you are there, even when he can't see you. And that makes life easier for both of you, especially when it comes to him learning to fall asleep, and back to sleep, by himself. Most psychologists agree that it isn't until a baby reaches around nine months old (but perhaps as young as seven months) that he grasps the notion of crying to get your attention. In this case, give reassurance according to whichever settling method you decide to follow (see pp86–93), and begin to listen out for the differences in his cries – there may be some that you don't need to respond to instantly (see p41). By the time he approaches a year old, you will be able to distinguish cries of pain, illness, or distress, and those of attention, or of "winding down" – and will respond appropriately.

What happens if I'm too tired to be consistent?

It's doubtful there is a parent in the land who, having set in place a sleep routine, hasn't let this slip at one time or another just to get some sleep. Don't be too hard on yourself, get a good night's sleep and then get back on track as quickly as possible. Feeling less tired will re-affirm your resolve. Refer to your list (see p15), and keep in mind the end goal – a lifetime of good sleep for all of you.

I'm worried about my baby waking other people

If you are concerned about your baby disturbing the sleep of your partner or other children – or the neighbours – try to find practical solutions. Could your baby sleep away from an adjoining wall? Children are generally deep sleepers, and get used to peripheral noise, but you could encourage older children to sleep with their door closed. If your baby and older child share a room, some disturbance may be inevitable. Starting their bedtime routines at different times so that one is asleep before the other can help each to settle down. And deal with any night waking with the minimum of fuss to limit the disturbance. As for your partner, a good pair of earplugs may be the answer!

My plan isn't working – what can I do?

The best of plans might prove impractical. Work out where it's going wrong – and make a new more suitable plan, then stick to that. A change in tactics doesn't mean you'll never get it right.

Focus on twins

Should my twins sleep together?
Co-bedding – putting babies in the same sleeping space – is perfectly safe and helps twins feel secure. They are more likely to regulate their sleeping cycles when together, although, generally, one will sleep through the cries of the other (so as they get older, don't necessarily rush to quieten the one who is fussing). If you do wish to help synchronize their rhythms, when one twin wakes for a night feed, but not the other, try waking the other for a feed, too, so you have some hours when both babies are fed and sleeping. Follow the same safe sleeping advice as for single babies (see p23). If co-bedding doesn't seem to be working for your twins, sleeping next to each other in separate cribs gives each the space to sleep contentedly, knowing the other is there.

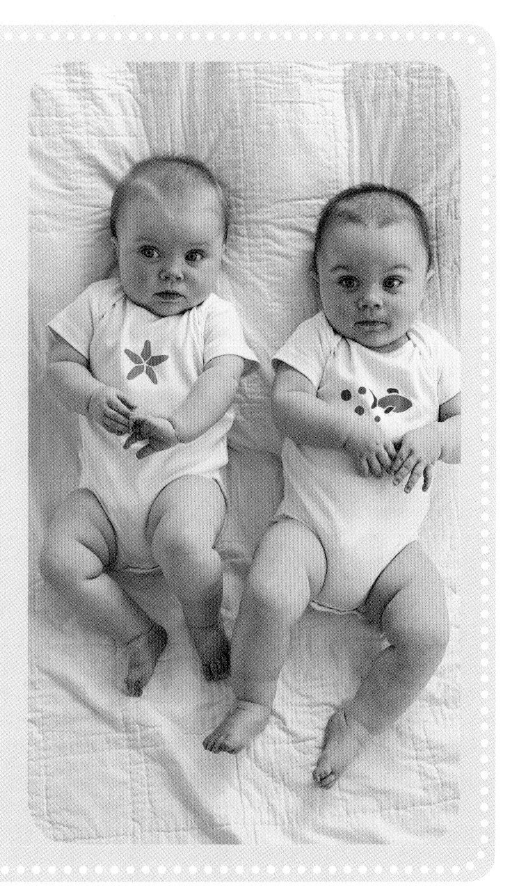

The sleeping parent

Your baby's happiness, and, indeed, that of your whole family, in no small part depends upon your own wellbeing: a happy parent makes for a happy baby. Spotting the signs of your own sleep debt and finding ways to repay it, even just a little, is good for you and your baby.

Signs of sleep debt

The most common sign of sleep debt is waking feeling unrefreshed. You may feel foggy and uncoordinated, be irritable and impatient, and find it hard to concentrate. Being tired can also lead to poor dietary choices as your body looks for a quick fix, often in the form of sugar, to improve energy levels. If you reach for sweets, chocolates, and biscuits more than you used to, you probably aren't getting enough sleep.

Research has shown that the more tired a new mother becomes, the more susceptible she is to postnatal depression. In fact, either parent may begin to feel sad, tearful, and generally unable to cope once they rack up a sleep debt.

Have you tried?

Expressing your milk. If lack of sleep is affecting how you cope in the day, consider expressing a couple of nighttime feeds each week so your partner can take a nightshift. Make the most of those nights: sleep in another room or wear earplugs so you have a chance to catch up on your sleep debt.

What can you do?

A recent study in West Virginia, USA, revealed that most new mothers who nap during the day, in general, still felt unrefreshed. However, there was good reason – their naps were not long enough or deep enough to be of any benefit. When you are suffering from sleep debt, try to make your naps longer – 90 minutes to two hours. This way you will go through a full sleep cycle (see p11), making the sleep more worthwhile. When your baby has a daytime nap, don't be tempted to do chores; instead, set an alarm for two hours' time, so that you don't have to worry about waking up, and sleep yourself.

If you find it hard to nap in the day, try to find some quiet time simply to relax.

Here are some ways to look after yourself:

• Make sure you sit down and rest – often. Being still, but not necessarily asleep, is almost as restful for your body as sleep itself. Don't undervalue those hours spent gazing at your new baby – they are good for you!

• Eat three meals and two snacks a day and keep them healthy. Oats, muesli, or wholemeal toast with a poached egg make a good breakfast that will set you up for the day, releasing energy slowly into your bloodstream so that you don't feel the need for a quick fix. A piece of fruit or some nuts make for healthy snacks. Steer clear of refined sugar and foods high in saturated fats.

• Release tension in your body. Sit or lie down and tense and release each of your muscle groups in turn, beginning with the soles of your feet and working up through your legs, torso, arms, hands, shoulders, neck, and head. As you release, feel the tension ebbing away.

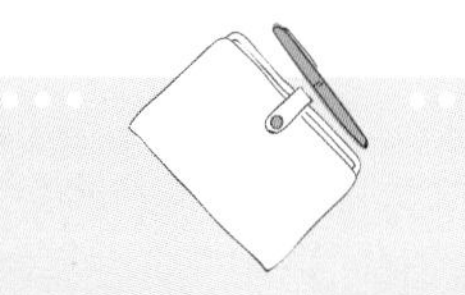

Coping at work

Of course, it's not always possible to nap in the day, especially if you are back at work. Follow the guidelines for healthy eating, left, to keep energy levels stable, and stay hydrated, drinking a glass of water every hour or so. In general, avoid sugary or caffeinated drinks, but you can have a strategic cup of coffee to counter energy dips – not more than two cups a day, and not later than three in the afternoon, though.

Schedule meetings for times when you feel most alert (perhaps first thing, or straight after lunch when your energy levels are higher). Keep your workspace well-ventilated and a little on the cool side, and take regular breaks, around every two hours, to walk around for a few minutes, ideally outside.

• Try a breathing exercise. Sit comfortably, close your eyes, and breathe in through your nose, deep into your diaphragm. At the top of an inhalation, make an "o" shape with your lips and slowly breathe out through your mouth. Repeat a few times, but stop if you feel dizzy.

• Try to make time each week for an activity that relaxes you and makes you feel good, whether running, dancing, singing, or having a bubble bath. Feel-good hormones released while doing something you love can help overcome negativity associated with tiredness.

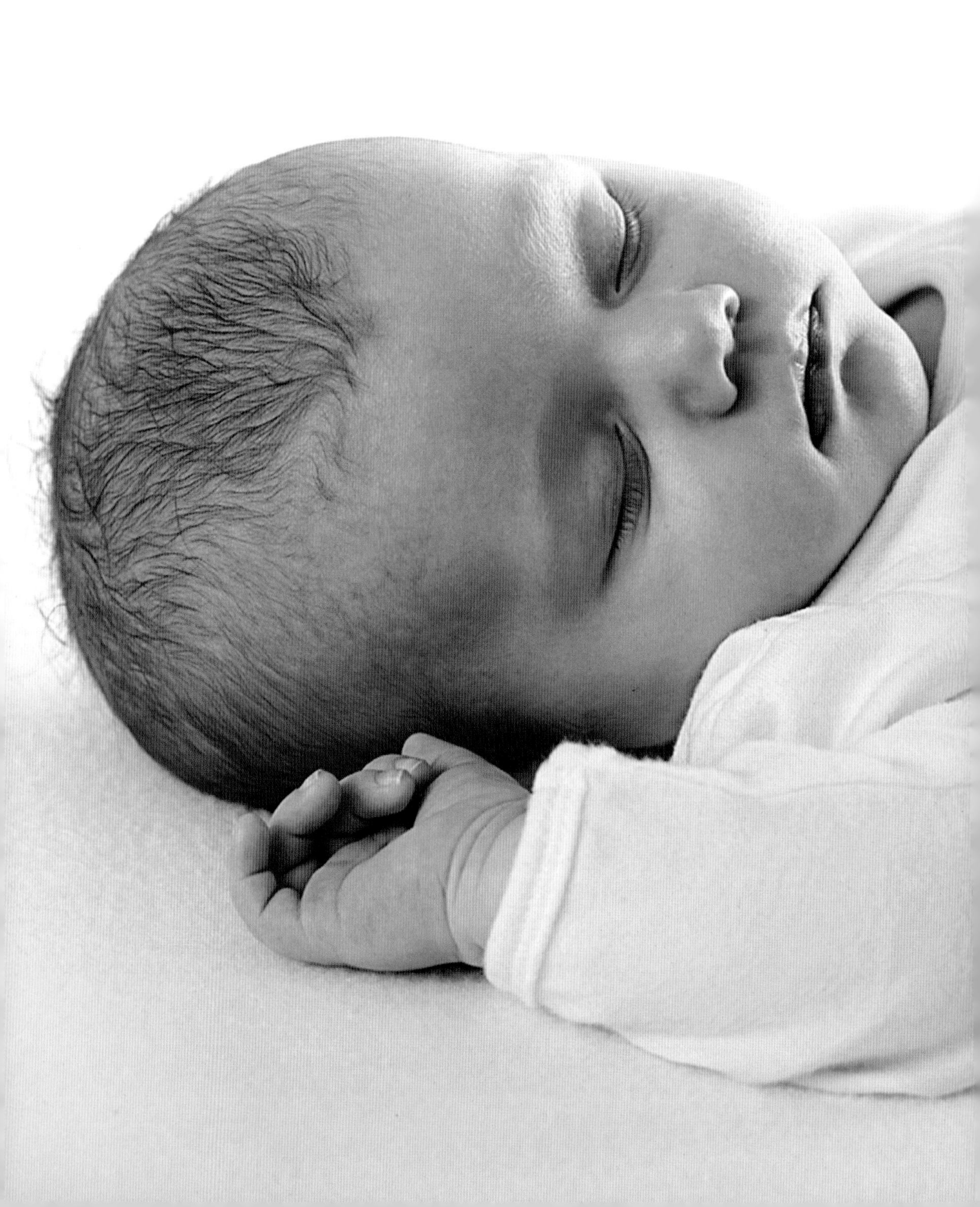

2

Newborns

The first few weeks with a new baby are often a bit of a blur. It is perfectly normal for parents to feel they have lost their own nighttime sleep, and for night and day to become one long period of naps, with waking interludes for feeding (both parents and baby) and socializing. Don't expect too much of yourself or your baby in these early weeks – take each day (and night) as it comes, and be as kind to yourself as possible. If family or friends offer to cook meals or to do your washing, thank them profusely and accept; if they want to visit and you're too tired, politely tell them so. Most of all, savour every moment of this unique time with your tiny baby. It will soon be over and better sleep for you all is just round the corner.

Where your baby sleeps

Your baby is not yet able properly to regulate her body temperature, and her breathing and heart rate can seem erratic. For these reasons, human babies thrive when kept close to their mothers. It's recommended that for the first six months of life, the safest place for your baby to sleep is in a Moses basket, crib, or cot in your room. If you prefer to co-sleep, you will need to follow guidelines (see below) to ensure your baby sleeps safely.

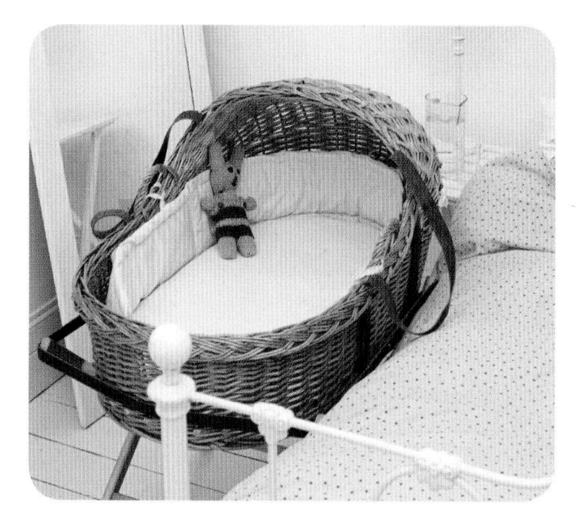

Moses baskets and cribs

While you can start off with your baby in a full-sized cot, a newborn can seem quite lost in one, and many parents opt for a cosier Moses basket or crib. The great benefit of a Moses basket is that your baby can move around with you. Recent research into reducing the incidence of cot death (Sudden Infant Death Syndrome, or SIDS; see box, opposite) suggests that the principle of keeping your baby in the same room as you while she sleeps should apply as much to daytime naps as it does to nighttime sleep.

Whatever sleeping space you use for your baby, try to make sure there's room for her to stretch her arms above her head and to the sides without touching the edges. Babies often make jerky movements during their sleep and knocking their knuckles against the sides of a crib or Moses basket can startle them awake.

Co-sleeping

In many cultures, families sleep together in one place, drawing comfort and security from being together. Co-sleeping, sharing your bed with your baby, has many practical benefits. If you are breastfeeding, having your baby next to you in the night enables her to latch on with the least disturbance to your, your partner's, or her own sleep. Studies also show that mothers tend to breastfeed for longer (that is, until the baby is older) than those who don't co-sleep. Your newborn is at her most insecure in those first few weeks, and sleeping in contact with

Don't co-sleep if you (or your partner) have drunk alcohol, taken drugs, have smoked, or are extremely tired.

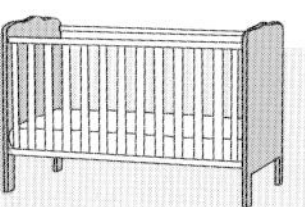

Safe sleeping

Sudden Infant Death Syndrome (SIDS) occurs when a baby suddenly stops breathing during sleep. We still don't fully understand what causes it, but there are certain guidelines that can help minimize the risks to your baby. Studies show that there is a dramatic reduction in risk if your baby sleeps in the same room as you until she is six months old. Putting your baby to sleep on her back is also thought to minimize the risk, as is arranging bedding so that your baby sleeps with her feet at the bottom of the cot ("feet to foot"). That way, if she wriggles down, she can't go beneath the covers. Keep toys, pillows, and bumpers out of the cot or sleeping space; and use cotton sheets and cellular blankets, safely tucked in. Avoid baby duvets or pillows until at least one year of age.

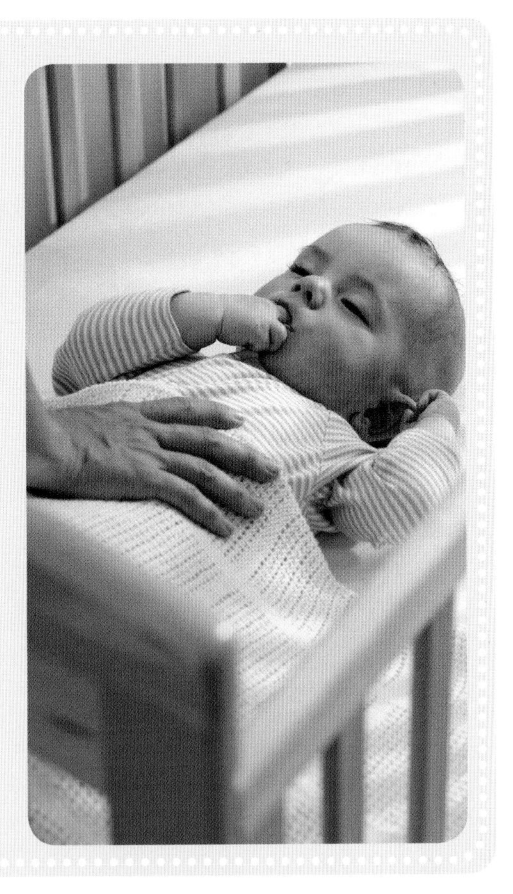

you and in a place where she can still hear your heartbeat may help her feel safe. Some also believe it helps the bonding experience.

However, having your baby in your bed may disturb your sleep, your baby's sleep, and your partner's sleep. Some experts believe co-sleeping should be avoided under three months of age as your baby could overheat dangerously. If you co-sleep, it's important that there are no pillows near your baby and that you don't use a duvet. Co-sleeping isn't recommended if your baby was premature or had a low birthweight. Never fall asleep on a sofa with your baby.

Your baby's bedding

Your baby can't yet self-regulate her temperature, so a cotton sheet with cellular blankets allows you to add and remove layers according to the room temperature. Tuck in the sides and bottom ends of all the bedding so your baby doesn't get tangled up if she moves. Bear in mind that a baby's hands often feel cold as her circulation isn't fully developed. Put two fingers on her chest (slip them under her sleepsuit), or on the back of her neck, and see how warm these areas feel: if they are cold, add a layer; if warm, even if her extremities feel chilly, she's fine.

Sleep cycles

While adults have sleep cycles that last roughly 90 minutes each, taking you through drowsy, to light, to deep, to dreaming sleep in four distinct stages, usually during a single, long sleep of about eight hours in the night, the sleep cycle of your newborn is dramatically different. Understanding the differences helps to explain why your baby disrupts your own sleep over the first few weeks of her life.

Newborn sleep cycles

Your newborn baby sleeps for around 16 hours in every 24, however, her sleep pattern is broken into lots of shorter sleeps over the course of the day and night, described as "polyphasic" sleep. Furthermore, whereas the phases of an adult's sleep vary over the course of the night, with periods of restful sleep decreasing, and of dreaming sleep increasing with each full cycle of sleep, a newborn baby's sleep is more or less evenly split between restful and dreaming sleep. The increased time spent dreaming is thought to be because it's possibly during dreaming sleep that your baby processes all the new information she receives every day – although no one knows for sure if this is the case.

It's best, in the early days, simply to adapt to your baby's sleep pattern.

For babies, restful sleep is generally linear – unlike an adult's periods of restful sleep, which are subdivided into phases of drowsy, light, and deep sleep – and each sleep cycle is between only 45 and 60 minutes long (compared with your 90 minutes). Your baby will go through only two or three sleep cycles (sometimes fewer) in each period of sleep, waking every two to three hours for food.

What all of this tells us is that it is perfectly normal and natural for your newborn baby to wake frequently during the night in the early weeks of life. In turn, this means that any form of sleep training before six weeks of age is likely to become a drain on your energies, and frustrating and unsettling for both of you – with little or no positive effect. Rather than trying to instil a strict routine now or attempting to teach your baby to self-soothe, in these very early stages of your new baby's life, it's best to go with her sleeping patterns and, in the meantime, do everything you can to preserve your own energy levels during the day.

Strategies for coping with broken nights

There are several practical strategies you can use to help you manage disturbed nights.

Claim back the sleep debt.
Read the information on napping and other ways to ease the load on pages 18–19. Try to get in at least one good nap every day. As well as daytime naps, go to bed earlier than you did before your baby was born: if your night is going to be broken, it's better to start it sooner.

Practise falling back to sleep easily during the night.
Create a little ritual for yourself that your mind will associate with falling back to sleep after you've fed or soothed your baby at night. It might be as simple as counting backwards from 300, or as elaborate as reciting your favourite poem to yourself, or visualizing yourself walking through a tranquil scene and conjuring up all the sights, sounds, and smells. Whatever it is, be consistent. Within a few nights, your mind should associate the ritual with falling asleep.

Help yourself to feel positive every day.
While for the first couple of weeks at least, you probably aren't aiming to do much apart from feed and tend to your baby, at some point you may start to fret about other jobs that need doing. Make a list of things you need to do and then put these in order of priority. Each day, focus on achieving only the first two or three items on the list – everything else can wait. Even if you manage only the first item, having actually seen something through from start to finish will help to stave off the sense of hopelessness that can come with sleep debt, keep things in perspective, and get jobs done – no matter how slowly.

Finally, remind yourself every day (and night) that it is a matter of only weeks before your baby will be ready to start to understand the notion of night and day, and from thereon you will be on a path back to a good night's sleep. Take heart – it's not for ever.

Setting up good sleep habits

Although your baby is still too little to understand, appreciate, or respond to sleep-training methods (see Chapter Seven), you can still begin, even from the earliest days, to get in to habits of good "sleep hygiene". This is the term that experts use to describe the environmental triggers and practices we have for going to sleep, including those we establish to separate night from day.

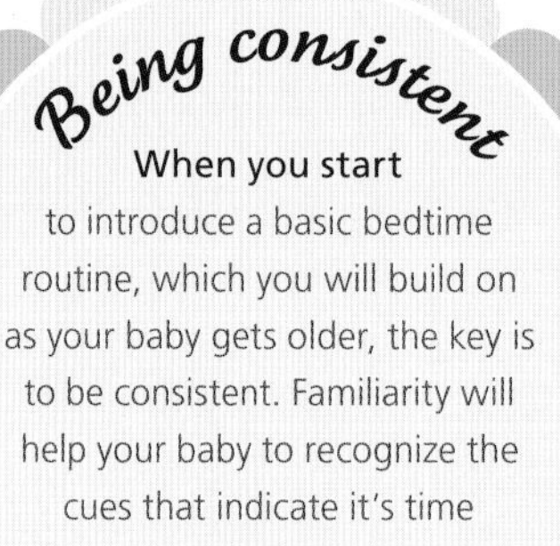

Being consistent

When you start to introduce a basic bedtime routine, which you will build on as your baby gets older, the key is to be consistent. Familiarity will help your baby to recognize the cues that indicate it's time to settle down for the night.

Nighttime triggers

Discuss with your partner when you think will be an appropriate bedtime for your baby once she is a little bit older, and particularly once she is sleeping in her own room. If this is your first baby, you might decide that 7pm is when you'll want her to settle down for the night; a second or subsequent baby may need to have a routine that begins a little earlier, to give you time to concentrate on your other children (see box, opposite).

Guidelines suggest that your baby sleeps in the same room as you until she reaches six months of age (see pp12–13), so the following first bedtime "routine" doesn't conclude with settling your baby down in her own room to sleep, but crucially it does introduce the notion of a separate day and night.

Winding down

An hour before your chosen bedtime for your baby, lower the lights in the house. If you don't have dimmer switches, position lamps with low-wattage bulbs in the rooms you use in the evening. In the summer months, draw some curtains or blinds to dim the light.

Give your baby a bath (or a "top and tail" clean with a flannel and cotton wool of her face, hands, body, and nappy area if you haven't started giving daily baths) and change her into a fresh sleepsuit, again within the hour before bedtime. Keep the lights low and your voice soft and calming. You could sing a bedtime song while she's in the bath or while dressing her for bed. Keep toys safely tucked away for the morning, and don't engage your baby in noisy or stimulating games. All of these little touches will become triggers for her that the mood has changed from one of light, noise, and activity, to a time of quiet rest.

When your baby is dressed, ready for "bed", try feeding her. Depending upon when she had her last feed, she may or may not be hungry, but even if she takes only a little milk, you're getting her into a routine of having a calming pre-bedtime feed. Wind her well, then put her in her Moses basket and rest yourself while she coos contentedly, and maybe even drops off. Of course, some babies, such as those with colic, may not settle easily. Carrying your baby close to you in a sling for a little while can help to soothe her before putting her down for the night.

Wake up, it's morning!

Understanding the difference between day and night is as much about noticing the contrast in the morning. When you are happy to start the day (bearing in mind that your baby will probably have been awake several times since midnight), open the curtains, or in winter turn on the lights. Now is the time for activity!

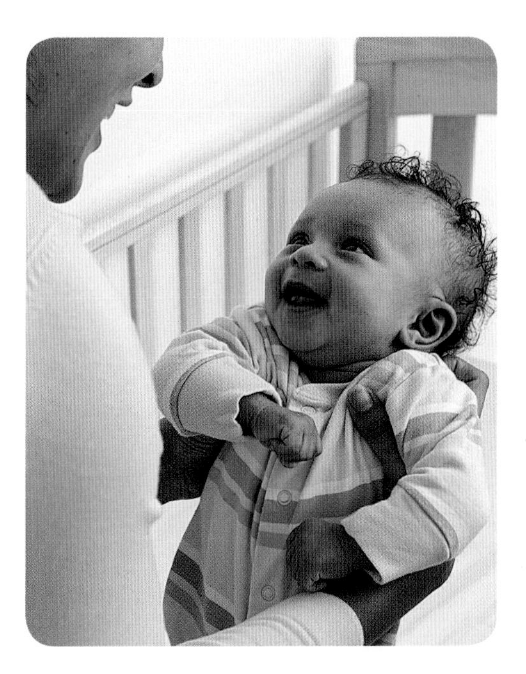

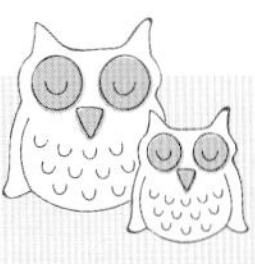

Sibling bedtimes

Introducing your newborn baby into a household where you already have a toddler poses its own challenges when it comes to bedtime. Most importantly, try not to change the routine that your toddler is used to. Around an hour or so before bedtime begins for your toddler, follow the bedtime sequence of events you have started to introduce for your baby, even if this seems too early in the evening. Remember that at this stage, you aren't trying to impose a routine on your baby, just introducing the notions of day and night and activity and rest.

Allowing your toddler to feel part of your baby's evening routine will help them both to bond; perhaps your toddler can help by passing you a nappy or new sleepsuit. Once your baby is bathed, calmed, and fed, there's a good chance that she will kick about contentedly in her Moses basket, allowing you to put your toddler to bed as normally as possible.

If your baby won't settle (and babies do have their own agendas at this young age), consider popping her into a sling so that you can carry her around with you. This will be soothing for your baby and allow you to devote both hands to your toddler, as well as much of your attention.

Soothing techniques

Your baby will learn to settle herself to sleep when a little older, but in the first few weeks, she may need your help – which is where soothing techniques come in. If these consistently don't work, talk to your health visitor.

Swaddling

Lay out a blanket, then bring the diagonally opposite corners together. Lay your baby face up on the blanket, her shoulders above the folded edge. Fold her left arm by her side, then fold the left side of the blanket over her shoulder and body, tucking the end under her. Repeat on the other side so she's snugly (but not tightly) bundled up. Don't swaddle after six weeks as it may be restricting.

Make "white noise". A washing machine can imitate the swooshing

Rocking

While she was in your womb, your baby moved around when you did. Before she reaches six weeks old, holding your baby and gently rocking her to sleep will not spoil her. Or hold her tummy down over your forearm (support her head) and rub her back while rocking her. Keep movements gentle and calming rather than stimulating.

Try running your finger gently over your baby's brow and nose.

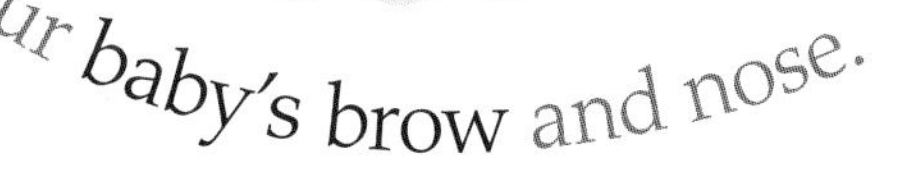

Side soothing

Experts believe that most toddlers sleep on their side with their knees slightly drawn up as this replicates the fetal position. Always put your baby to sleep on her back (see p23), but if she needs soothing, try supporting her on her side: watch her closely and if she settles, gently turn her onto her back.

Get moving

Most babies settle quickly when taken for a walk in their buggy, or for a short drive in their car seat – although if you do this often, your baby may grow to rely on it. During the day, put your baby in a sling so that she is permanently close to you and moves with you. Choose a sling you think will suit you both, perhaps a structured baby carrier-type sling, or a pouch-style sling with stretchy fabric.

sound of the womb.

Pacifiers

According to recent research, as well as providing comfort, a dummy may reduce the risk of SIDS (see p23). However, in the first four weeks it may discourage the impetus to breastfeed – it takes less effort to suck on a dummy than to draw milk from a nipple. Limit its use to nap- and bedtimes, and if it falls out during sleep, don't put it back.

Your baby's sleep environment

In the early weeks of life, your baby's sleep environment is mainly centred around her cot, crib, or Moses basket. However, the ambience of the room around her, as well as the light, temperature, and noise levels can all teach her good – or bad – sleeping habits, from her earliest days. Newborn babies are infinitely suggestible. The sleep-triggers you establish even from the very beginning can stay with your baby throughout her childhood (and even her life), helping her to fall asleep easily.

Setting the mood

When you put your baby down for a nap, draw the curtains or lower the lighting. At night, it's a good idea to get her used to sleeping without a nightlight (see box, opposite). Keep noise levels low, although you may want her to get used to sleeping with some background noise during the day. Loud or sudden noises that she can hear from her room may startle her, whereas some gentle music can be soothing, as can monotonous "white" noise, such as the hum of the washing machine, which replicates the sound of the womb. If you've other children at home, keep the mood calm by making your baby's naptimes an opportunity for some quiet games – story-telling or puzzles are perfect.

Regulating temperature

It's only once your baby reaches around two years of age that she will be able to regulate her temperature in the way that you do. Until then, it's important that her sleeping environment is

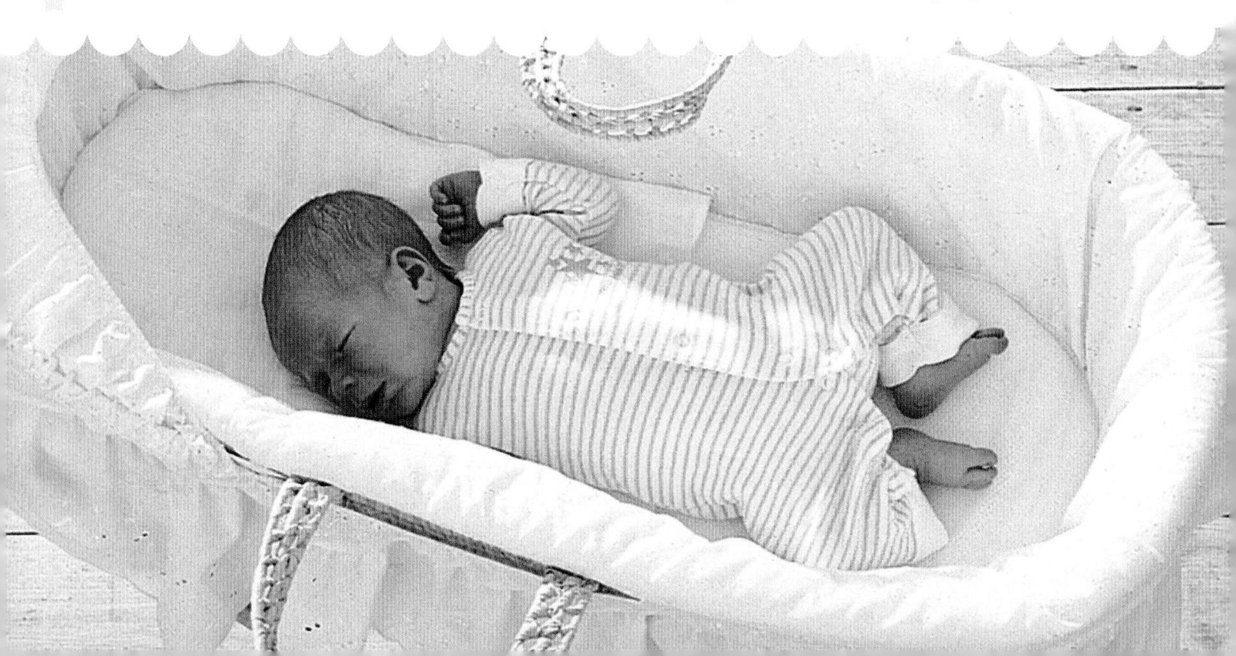

kept at as constant a temperature as possible. Experts recommend a room temperature of between 16 and 20°C (60.8 and 68°F), with 18°C (64.4°F) as ideal – neither too hot, nor too cold. However, if you're worried about your baby overheating, err on the side of caution and keep the room cooler, then add more layers of sheets and blankets in your baby's cot. Once she starts to wriggle, try a baby sleeping bag, which does up over her shoulders and will stop her shuffling free from her covers.

In warmer months, keep the curtains drawn throughout the day to stop the sun heating up the room. You could open an upper window to keep the room ventilated (but make sure that an older child couldn't climb out of it and also that your baby is not sleeping in a draught). Use fewer blankets, too.

Have you tried?

A red nightlight.

As darkness falls, the brain releases melatonin, triggering sleep. Some experts believe that nightlights hamper this process. If you need light, perhaps for a night feed, use a red bulb: the brain doesn't perceive red light as daylight, so it has little, or no, effect on melatonin secretion.

A soothing, comfortable environment is conducive to good sleep.

Sleeping on the move

Getting out and about with your baby is important, so it's useful to get her used to sleeping on the move. Before six months, your baby will need to lie flat in a buggy or pram, just as she does in her cot or crib, so make sure you can easily reposition her buggy seat to tilt into a more horizontal position, supporting her head and neck and keeping her spine in its natural curve. A hood keeps the sun or the rain off your baby's head, and will also help her feel more enclosed if you're trying to get her to sleep.

In winter months, a foot muff will keep tiny toes snug, while a sheepskin or fleece liner that goes on top of the seat for your baby to lie on, will help prevent the cold air coming in from the back. Always keep a hat, gloves, and extra blankets handy so that you can wrap her up warm, and a rain cover will help to keep out not only the rain, but the wind, too.

Finally, for the summer months it's worth investing in a universal buggy blackout blind that attaches to the buggy frame (and often a car seat) in the same way you attach a rain cover. Made from breathable fabrics, these keep out the sun's harmful rays, keep the buggy cool, and provide your baby with a cosy, dark space in which to sleep.

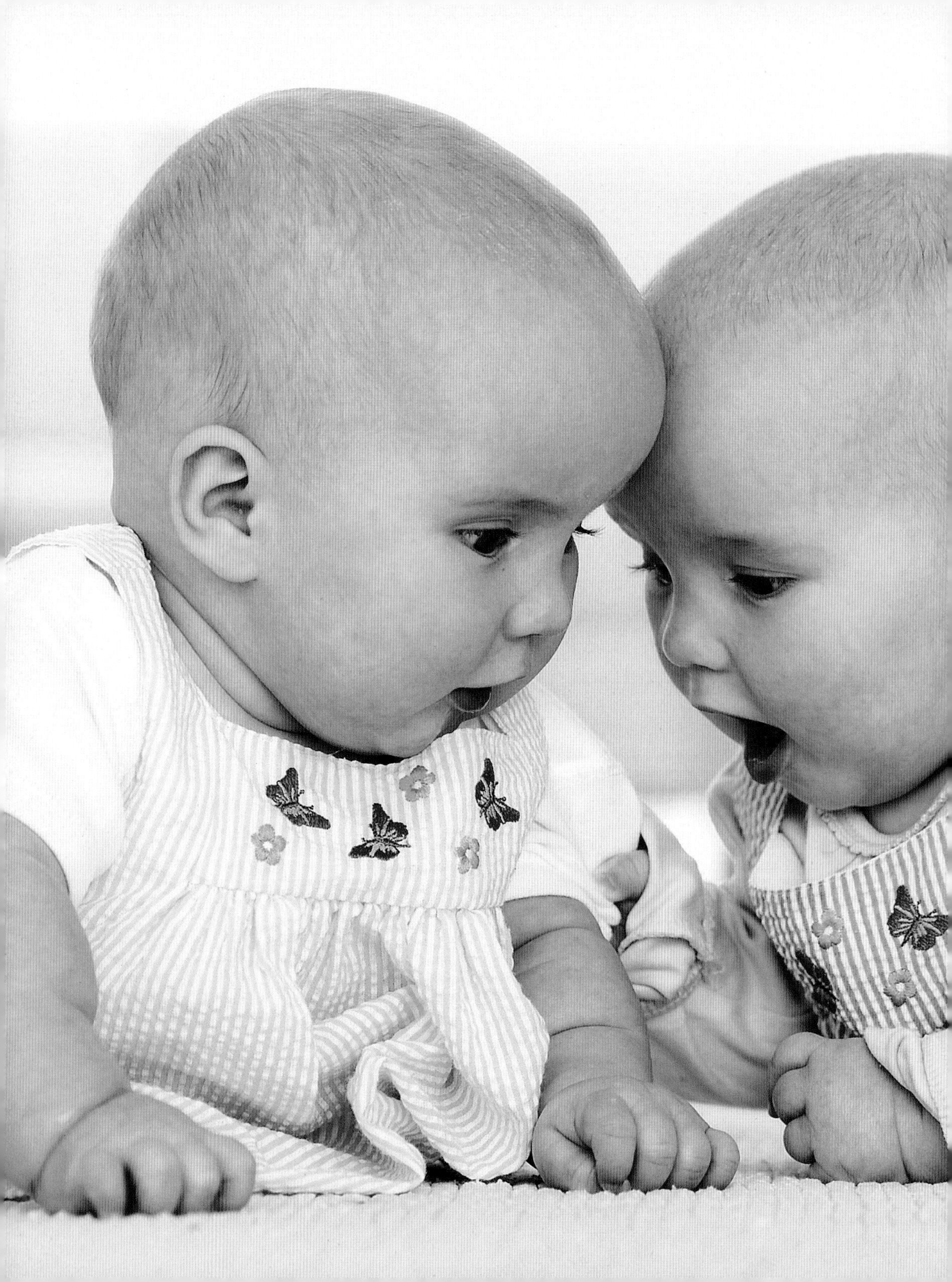

3

6 weeks to 6 months

The period from six weeks to six months old is one of rapid development for your baby. The newborn phase is over and she will start to settle into the routine of daily life. This is the time to capitalize on your baby's suggestibility, as habits that you establish now will be ones that can last her a lifetime. Also, happily for you, it's during this time that, with some commonsense and consistency, you could have your baby sleeping for longer periods through the night – and that means more nighttime sleep for you, your partner, and any other members of your family, too.

Where your baby sleeps

By six weeks old, your baby may be starting to outgrow his crib or Moses basket and it could be time to move him to a cot.

Choosing a cot

Consider whether you want a cot or a cot bed. Cots have fixed or drop-down sides and will last until your baby is around two years old, depending upon the size you buy. Cot beds, on the other hand, have removable sides. Being able to remove only one side will enable you to bring the cot right up against your own bed (as long as the base can be adjusted to match the exact height of your bed). This is a great choice if you want to co-sleep with your baby, but are worried about rolling over on top of him, or think your own bed is too small for two parents and a baby.

When you set up your baby's new cot, make extra sure all screws and bolts are securely fastened.

If you are considering a cot with a drop-down side, which makes it easier for you to lift your baby in and out, make sure it carries the necessary kite marks and safety certificates. Safety issues with some manufacturers have meant that cots with drop-down sides have been banned in the USA since 2011, although they are still available in Europe.

Cot beds have greater longevity because, once both sides are removed, they can convert into toddler beds. From your baby's point of view, this can make the transition from a cot to a "big bed" easier.

Have you tried?

A basket in a cot. When your baby has almost outgrown his Moses basket, try easing the transition to a big cot by putting the basket in the cot at first, allowing him to get used to the new environment more gradually.

Cot safety

Think carefully about the safety aspects of the cot you choose. Does it have an adjustable base so that you don't have to bend over too far to pick up your baby? Once he can pull himself up, at around nine months old, can you lower the base sufficiently that he couldn't launch himself over the side? Does the cot have a teething rail? Babies will gnaw against anything that might soothe sore gums and some cots come with a baby-safe plastic layer along the top bars. Finally, make sure the bars of the cot are not spaced too far apart – you don't want little legs or (worse) heads getting stuck; and check that fingers couldn't get caught in any drop-down or moving mechanism on the cot.

Finally, a cot on casters will enable you to move your baby from room to room if you need to. Make sure the wheels are lockable, though – once your baby gets to six months, he may well be wriggling about enough to move the cot around, too!

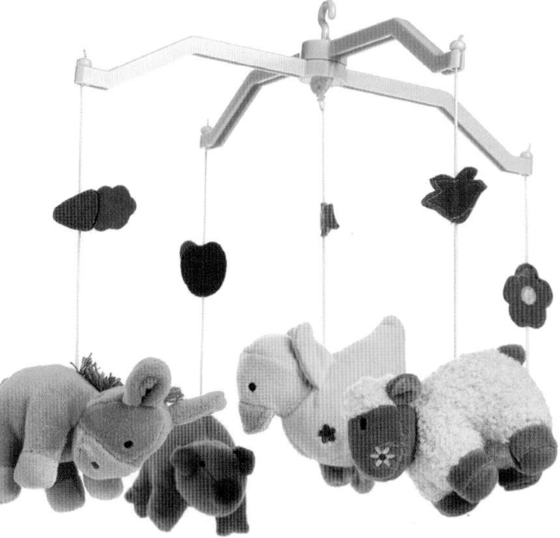

A mobile helps make the cot a happy place.

Choosing a mattress

The most important thing about your baby's mattress is that it fits the cot properly – make sure the measurements are compatible so that there are no gaps that your baby could get wedged into. Avoid second-hand or damp mattresses, too. It's worth buying a mattress with a removable, washable cover, in case of leaky nappies, or posseting. And as with your mattress, your baby's should be firm enough to support the natural curve of his spine.

Bedding

Your baby's cot bedding should tuck under the sides of the mattress to keep him feeling secure as well as snug. Use layered sheets and blankets, and avoid bumpers and soft toys in the cot, which pose a suffocation risk.

Cot toys

Once your baby is close to six months old, you might like to attach a special cot toy to the sides of his sleeping space, or a colourful mobile above it. These are great for making the cot a positive, happy place, but bear in mind that you want him to associate his cot with sleeping. Nonetheless, if, for example, you need to be able to put your baby in a safe place while you attend to a sibling, a cot toy might be just the thing to keep him occupied. You could always remove the toy at bedtime, or once he's asleep.

Daytime naps

Over the course of these first months, your baby will begin to sleep longer at night and have more regular naps during the daytime (see p36). Guidelines suggest that babies sleep in the same room as you during both nighttime and daytime sleeps. As your baby is outgrowing his Moses basket around now, think how you can provide a safe napping environment in the same room as you. You might be able to use his buggy, or invest in a travel cot, which you can easily put up and down according to where you are in the house. Or use your baby's naptime as the perfect excuse to catch up on some sleep in your own bed.

Sleep cycles

At some point before six months of age, your baby will begin to sleep for longer stretches of time during the night, waking for only one or two feeds (rather than three or four). Even though his tummy still isn't big enough to keep him going for a full eight hours just yet, he's reaching a point at which the amount of sleep you all get takes a turn for the better.

How much sleep?

In general, over the course of this time your baby will sleep for around 15 hours in every 24. Many experts believe that 10 of those hours can, by five or six months of age, happen at night, with the remaining five being made up of three daytime naps – typically a short morning nap, a longer lunchtime nap, and a short teatime nap.

Don't expect too much too soon, though – every baby is different. Try not to get frustrated if you think your baby's sleep doesn't seem to be following the pattern set out by experts. Instead, learn to recognize your baby's signs of sleepiness and respond to them, while at the same time continuing to establish the triggers that will become your baby's bedtime routine. Eventually, your baby will get the hang of the fact that the day is for playing and the nighttime for sleeping.

Changes to your baby's sleep cycle

Although your baby's sleep cycle (see p11) won't reach the full 90 minutes until about four years of age, during his first few months of life it becomes increasingly less likely that he'll wake fully during the brief periods of wakefulness when one sleep cycle ends and the next one

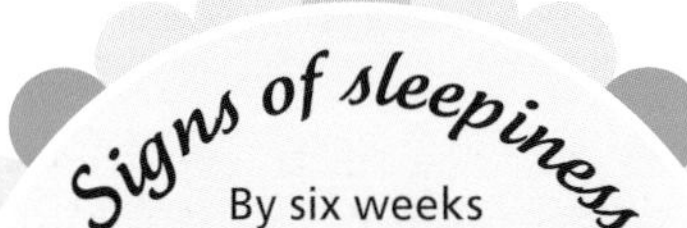

Signs of sleepiness

By six weeks old, your baby will show signs when he's sleepy. Each baby is different, but some common clues are:

- being fidgety or agitated (but has a clean nappy and isn't hungry)
- pulling at or rubbing his ears
- rubbing his eyes
- gazing ahead.

Whereas at birth your baby's sleep cycle was split roughly 50:50 between periods of REM and of non-REM sleep, as the six-month mark approaches, the amount of time your baby spends in dreaming sleep starts to fall off slightly, with periods of non-REM sleep gradually increasing. Non-REM sleep in adults is made up of three distinct phases: drowsy, light, and deep sleep. At birth, your baby had linear non-REM phases, with no fluctuations in sleep depth, but as periods of this type of sleep start to lengthen, his sleep depth slowly starts to fluctuate, too.

begins. This is probably because he can go for longer stretches now without a feed, even if he still can't manage to go the whole night. You will also have started to teach him the difference between night and day.

Over time, your baby will begin to settle more easily when he wakes in the night.

Each of your baby's sleep cycles is still made up of REM (dreaming) sleep and periods of non-REM sleep. You may be able to tell when he is dreaming because his eyes will move quickly, flickering beneath his eyelids – hence the name Rapid Eye Movement – and his arms and legs might twitch. Before six weeks, these jerky movements might have startled him awake fully, but now he is more likely to sleep through them.

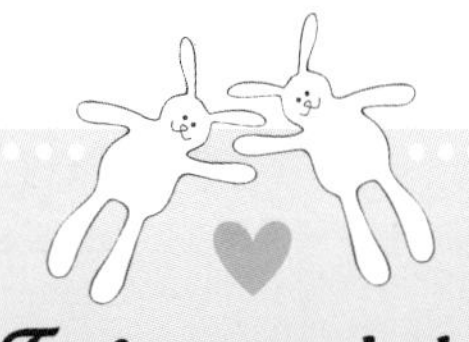

Twins and the unbroken night

Many sleep experts believe that a baby's ability to sleep through the night has less to do with chronological age and more to do with development and weight. As twins tend to have a lower birthweight (or at least one twin does), it may take longer for them to become good nighttime sleepers. Don't force the process: between six weeks and six months, twins – just like other babies – will start to sleep through, waking only for one or two feeds. It just may take a bit longer for twins than singletons. The good news is that, usually, twins start to sleep through at the same time.

Setting up good sleep habits

At six weeks of age, your baby is ready to make some progress with learning the difference between day and night and settling into a more regular bedtime routine. The little rituals you set in place now will become cues for sleeptime as he grows older.

Reinforcing your baby's bedtime routine

During the first few weeks of your newborn's life, you may have already begun to establish a rudimentary routine (see pp26–7). Now that your baby is old enough to begin to appreciate the pattern you've put in place, you can start to add to it. Although he may not respond to these bedtime prompts immediately, his rapid rate of learning between six weeks and six months means that he will pick up the cues soon enough. Here are some ideas of what you might incorporate into a bedtime routine to mark the transition from day to night.

• Sing the same lullaby to your baby each evening, perhaps while you're giving him his bedtime feed, bathing him, or dressing him for bed. Sounds are some of the earliest cues your baby will learn to understand, and your voice is already very soothing to him.

• Read a bedtime story. Although your baby may be too little to turn the pages or understand the words yet, he can still enjoy the soothing sound of your voice and the rhythm of the words.

• Say goodnight to a favourite teddy – this can make a great bedtime ritual. When your baby

Wake-up call

A regular wake-up time helps to set your baby's body clock. Gently wake him around the same time each day, opening curtains or blinds to let in the light. If he wakes earlier, don't rush to pick him up: encourage him to lie quietly until you get up. Then, except for nap times, make the day full of activity and interaction.

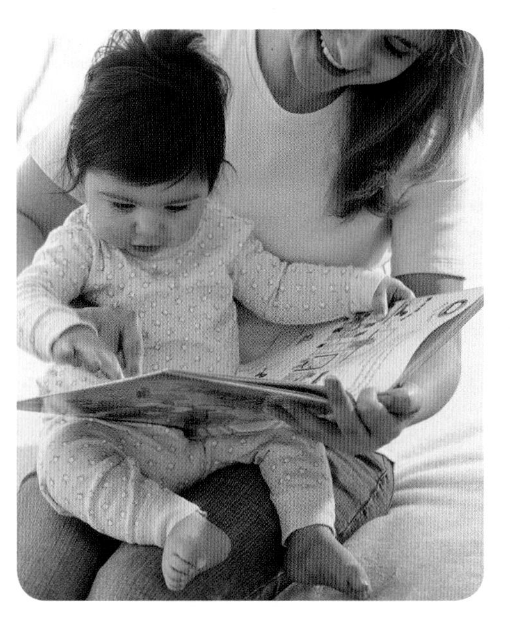

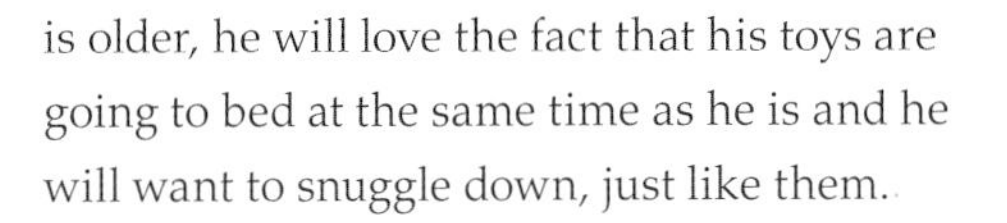

is older, he will love the fact that his toys are going to bed at the same time as he is and he will want to snuggle down, just like them.

Nighttime feeds

The last part of your bedtime routine will probably be your baby's evening feed. Make sure you're both comfortable, keep the lights low, and try not to engage with him too much. The point is to get him used to the idea that daytime is for talking and eye contact and evenings are quiet and less social.

Experts suggest that you try to avoid your baby falling asleep during this feed, partly so he doesn't stop eating before he's full (which will make him more likely to wake in the night hungry), but also so that you can put him to bed while he is drowsy, but still awake. This will help him to learn to ease himself off to sleep without thinking he needs to be in your arms. If it's hard to keep your snoozy baby awake for the whole feed, try gently stroking his cheek or shifting your position if he is nodding off. When he has finished his milk, lower him into his cot, or other sleeping space, say goodnight quietly, and leave the room.

During the evening, gradually wind down your baby's activities, so that he is calm and ready to settle.

If your baby wakes in the night, keep the lights low (see pp30–1), then feed, comfort, or change him according to his needs, but, again, try not to interact with him.

Going back to work

If you intend to go back to work – whether that's soon or in a year's time, it's a good idea to put in place right from the start routines that are most likely to be compatible with your working life. Think about:

- **What time you'll return** home from work. If you are working usual office hours, would that mean that you would rather your baby's bedtime was a little later than might seem ideal now to give you some additional precious time together? In which case, would you be happy for him to have a late-afternoon nap, say, around 5pm? However, do look out for signs of him being overtired, such as excessive crankiness, or increased nighttime restlessness, and consider whether you would have better quality time together, even for less time, if he went to bed a little earlier.

- **What time you'll need** to get to work in the morning. Would it make more sense for you to get up and shower while your baby is sleeping, rather than trying to occupy him while you get ready? In which case, resist picking him up as soon as he wakes, and encourage him to occupy himself in his cot for half an hour to give you time to get ready. Or organize a morning rota with your partner so you both have time to get ready while the other does the babycare.

Self-settling

One of the greatest things you can do for your baby (and by extension yourself) is to encourage him to self-settle. This is when he puts himself to sleep – or back to sleep – without needing any interaction with you.

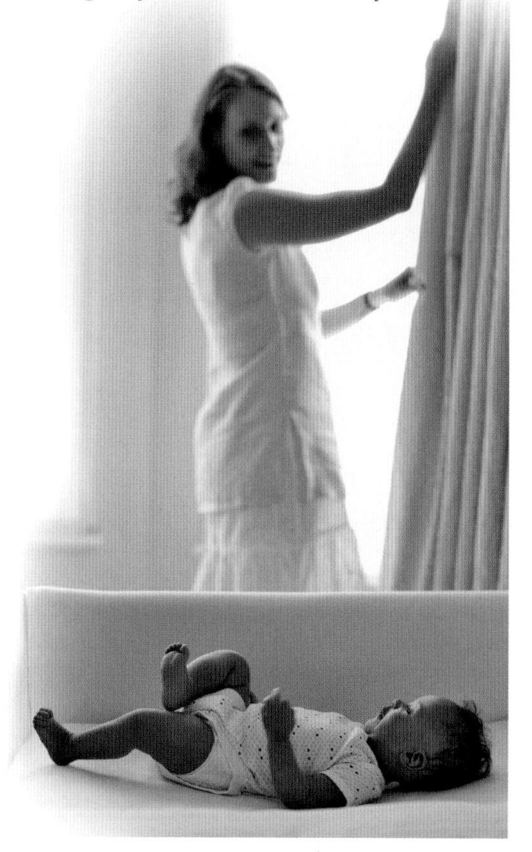

Strategies for self-settling

Most babies are more or less ready to learn to fall asleep on their own at six to eight weeks old. Even if your baby doesn't respond straight away, this is a good time to start to introduce the notion that he won't always need to fall asleep in your arms. If your baby is colicky, self-settling may have to wait a little longer and you will need to continue to use the soothing techniques from the early weeks (see pp28–9).

Learning to fall asleep on his own will serve your baby well for the years ahead.

To help your baby self-soothe, put him down to sleep while he is drowsy, but still awake. In the daytime, look for his sleepy signs (see p37) and as soon as you spot any, change him into a fresh nappy, dim the lights or draw the curtains, minimize any noise, and place him on his back in his sleeping space. At night, follow your bedtime routine, remembering to stop him falling asleep during his last feed (see p39), then put him down as usual.

Decide before you put this into practice what you will do once your baby is in his cot – will you say a soft "night night" and leave the room straight away? Or whisper "shhh...", stay for a few moments and then leave; or maybe you will decide that you want to stay in the room so that your baby can sense your presence close by until he's completely asleep.

Whatever you decide, bear in mind that it's often easiest to begin as you mean to go on, and be consistent in your approach. That applies to anyone else who puts your baby to bed, too.

Dealing with fussing

It's likely that your baby will fuss a little bit when you first put him in his cot, particularly at the start of his daytime nap. Calmly soothe him with "shhh..." sounds or gentle pats, and try to settle him without lifting him up. If this doesn't work and he begins to get distressed, pick him up and give him a cuddle until he's calm, then try again – repeating the ritual of putting him in his bed and tucking him in in exactly the same way as before. Consistency is key!

Using comforters

For some babies, it's less the being in someone's arms and more the comfort that comes with sucking during a feed that makes it so easy to fall asleep. If you seem to have a particularly "sucky" baby, consider using a dummy. The dummy will probably fall out once your baby is asleep, in which case take it out of his bed rather than pop it back in. That way, when he wakes briefly between sleep cycles he will learn to go back to sleep without his dummy in his mouth.

If you think a toy or comfort blanket might reassure him, make sure that there is no danger that he could get tangled up in it, or smother himself with it. Consult your health visitor, but as a general rule, once your baby is able to pull himself up or manoeuvre himself around, he is safe to have a comforter.

Use the comforter, or dummy, only at nap- and bedtimes, though, so that your baby associates it only with going to sleep – and so that you don't have to carry it around with you wherever you go.

Give sleep a chance

Finally, if your baby wakes during the night and you can hear him snuffling, give him a chance to put himself back to sleep before you soothe him or let him know you're near.

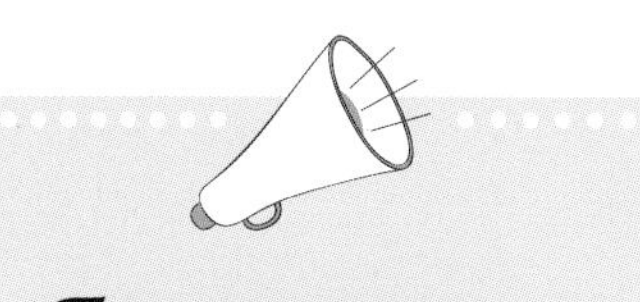

The language of crying

Now that your baby is getting older, he'll have developed different cries for communicating his different emotions or needs. For example, he might complain-cry if he has a wet or dirty nappy; cry in a yawny sort of a way when tired; and make a cry that's more guttural or strangulated if he is in pain or unwell. He will probably also have a certain cry when he just wants your attention.

Trust your instinct as you learn to decipher this language of crying. Use your baby's routine to help you with the decoding: if your eight-week-old hasn't had a feed for three hours, he is likely to be hungry; if he has been awake and stimulated for two or three hours, he is probably tired; if it's been four hours since his last fresh nappy, perhaps he needs a change. As you work out your baby's meanings, you'll have more confidence in deciding when it's okay to leave him to cry for a bit, and when he has a need that you should attend to.

Growth spurts

Just at the point where your baby appears to be making good progress with sleeping, and nights are more consistent, he seems to take several steps backwards. Don't panic – it's likely that your baby is going through a growth spurt, a period when his weight and his length (or height when he's older) rapidly increase.

Your baby will have growth spurts at two to three weeks old, then at six

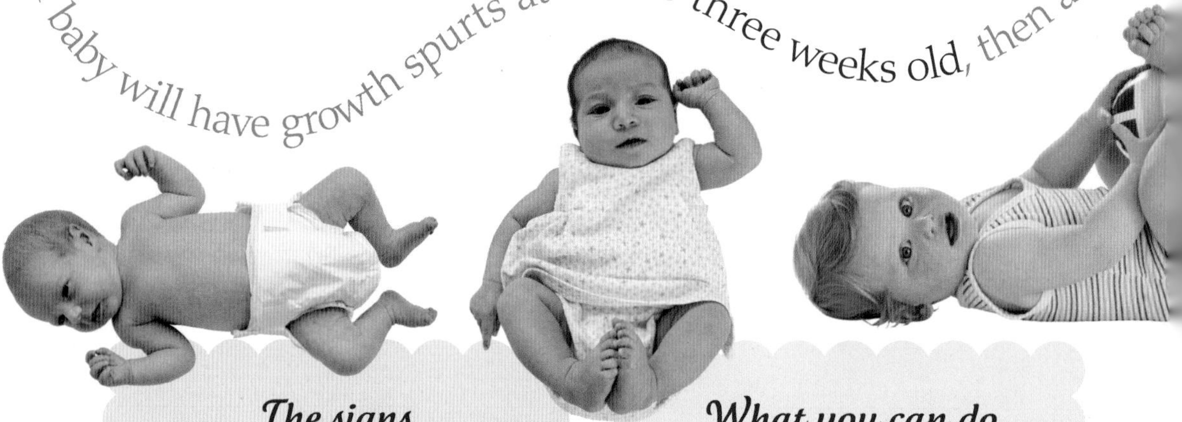

The signs

The confluence of certain aspects of your baby's life and behaviour make it likely that a growth spurt is in progress. First, growth spurts occur at certain ages (see above). Then, your baby may have an insatiable appetite. If you're breastfeeding, he may want to latch on all the time, and never be quite satisfied after a feed. He may be fussy or agitated, and may wake more at night, usually to feed, but maybe because growth hormones are most active during sleep, causing discomfort or agitation. (The jury's out as to whether there's such a thing as "growing pains".) Some babies sleep for longer periods in the day and are restless at night; others do the opposite. Usually, though, if sleep and feeding disruption come together, your baby's at an appropriate age, and isn't unwell, a growth spurt is the reason.

What you can do

Although having a fussy, hungry, and perhaps less restful baby can be unsettling for you, for your baby it is a normal part of development. Stick to your sleeping and waking routines, and try to hold your resolve with decisions on how to encourage him to self-settle. If he wants to feed more, you can be accommodating, but try not to let the feeding pattern you've established slip too much. If you're breastfeeding, encourage him to empty your breasts fully at each feed. This will have the effect of not only making sure he's getting the filling and sustaining hind-milk, but also will increase your milk production to meet the needs of your growing baby. If you're bottle-feeding, you may need to increase the amount you are giving at each feed by 25ml (1fl oz).

to eight weeks, three months, six months and nine months.

How you cope

Most of all, try not to worry about your baby. While it can be disconcerting when his behaviour changes, especially when he seems so unsettled, remind yourself that this is simply a natural part of his growth and development. If you're breastfeeding, stock up on healthy snacks so that you have the energy needed for increased milk production, and make sure you are drinking plenty of water to replace lost fluids. Reassure yourself that growth spurts – and the disruption they can cause – don't tend to last for more than a few days, so things should get back on track pretty quickly.

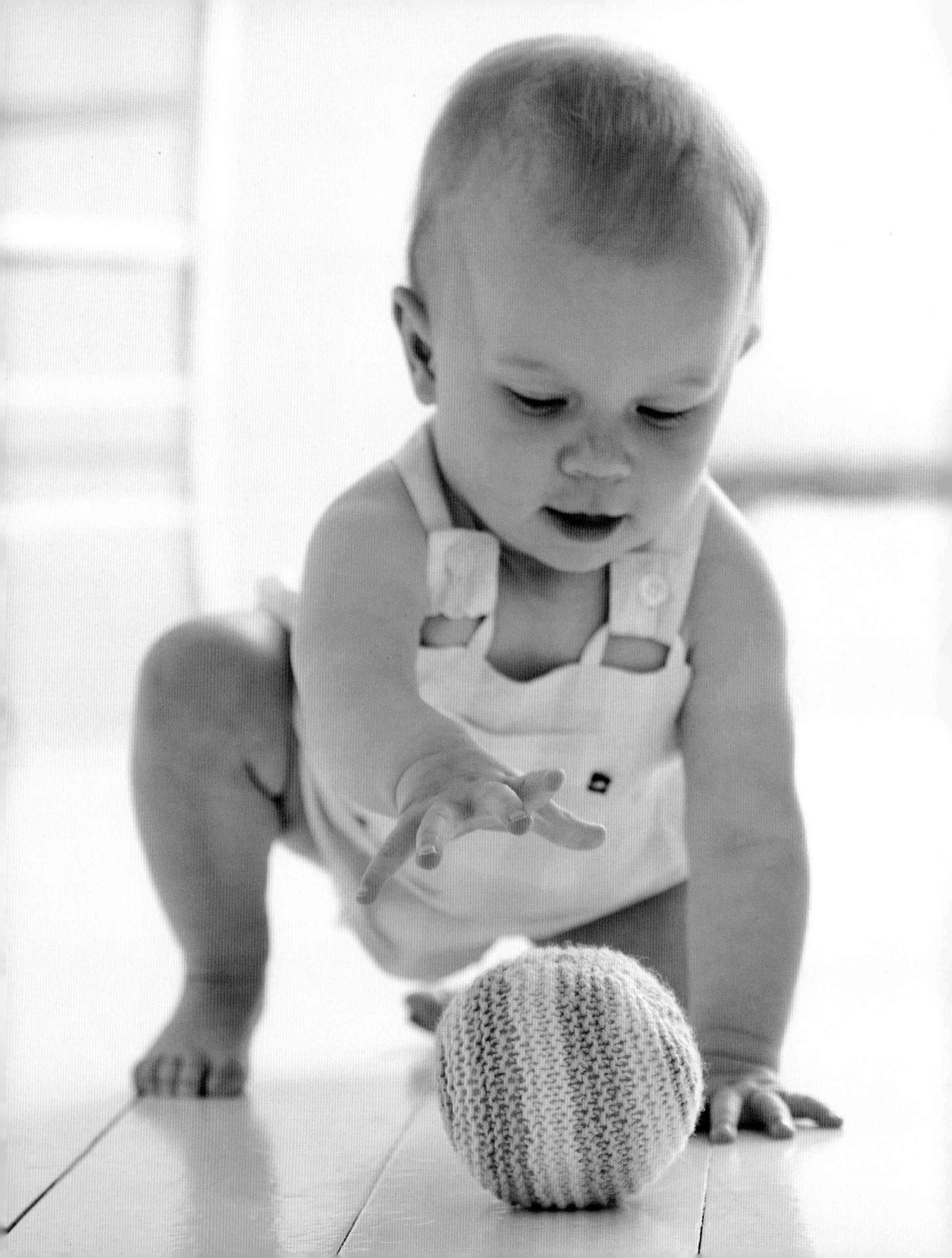

4

6 to 12 months

The second half of your baby's first year is a time of great change in her sleeping life. Not only will she probably move into her own bedroom, if she hasn't already, but she will also start to eat solid food. This should have the effect of making her less hungry at night and so more able to sleep through. She will also become aware enough to begin to make her demands on your time and attention at will. Many parents find this the most challenging time in the sleep story of their baby – as well as needing to hold your resolve to ensure your baby receives clear messages, you will now be six months into a cycle of broken nights yourself, and therefore at your most tired.

Where your baby sleeps

If your baby hasn't already moved out of your bedroom, or your bed, between six and 12 months will probably be the time when you start to consider settling her in to her own sleeping space.

Staying together

Not all babies are ready to move into their own room at six months. Follow your instincts: if you are all sleeping well as you are, you may decide to wait. Just be aware that babies younger than nine months tend to adapt more quickly. But you are the best judge of what suits your family.

A room of her own

Babies like routine, so the first thing to say about moving your baby into her own room is that it would be perfectly normal for her to have a few unsettled nights as she gets used to her new surroundings. Keep your eye on the goals: a lifetime of good sleep habits for your baby and better sleep for you. A little bit of disruption is perfectly normal and will pass.

Easing the transition

Keep to your routine. Stick to the bedtime you have set for your baby, and follow all the usual triggers that lead up to going to bed. In this way, only the place your baby sleeps in will change, minimizing the disruption to her life.

Second, consider whether you're going to go for a one-hit approach, moving her for naps and nighttime sleep all on the same day, or whether you might first consider putting her in her own room for her naptimes and then moving her in at night only once she is sleeping there happily during the day.

There may be other variables that can create stages in the process, too. For example, if your baby has been sleeping in a crib, small cot, or your bed until now and she is to have a new cot in her own room, you might consider moving the cot into your room for a few weeks before moving both the new cot and your baby into the separate room.

Take pleasure in creating a comfortable and inviting room for your baby.

Creating a sleepy space

Good sleep hygiene (see p26) includes creating a bedroom that is conducive to sleep.

• Keep your baby's room cooler rather than warmer, layering her up with blankets during the winter as needed, just as you have done since she was born. We fall asleep as our temperature falls most rapidly, so she will find it harder to drop off if the room is too warm.

• Use heavyweight curtains or blinds, or ideally blackout blinds, to make sure that your baby's room is dark whenever you settle her there for a sleep (see p30). (Open the curtains to let light in at the time you've set for waking up, too, of course.) Also consider whether you will leave on a nightlight or the landing light, which may be helpful if your baby isn't used to complete darkness.

• Decorate your baby's room in a calming colour – brighter walls covered in pictures may be too interesting and stimulating for her to settle easily to sleep. Soft blues, greens, pinks, and yellows work well.

• Try to ensure that her bedroom is a place of calming experiences – somewhere where you are always smiley and loving, and where you also always speak softly to her and give her cuddles. This will help her to associate her room with a soothing place where she can relax.

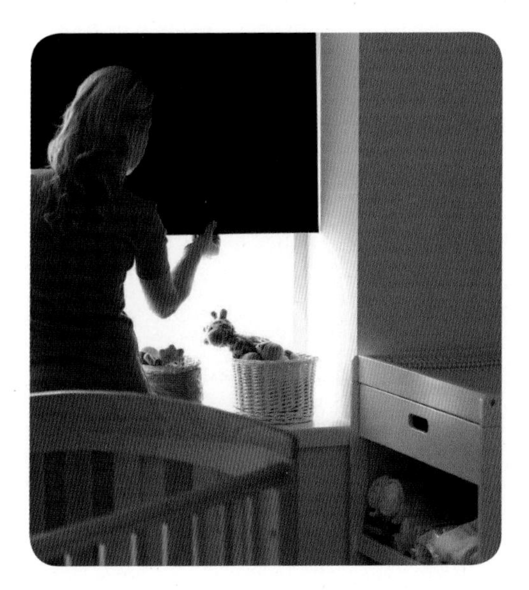

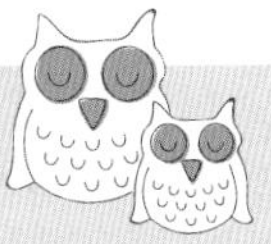

Sharing a room

By around six to nine months, most babies can go a full night without waking for a feed, so this may be a good time to move your baby into a room with siblings. Consider not only how well your baby is sleeping, but also how well your other children sleep. Most toddlers can sleep through inevitable baby noises, but older children might find it more difficult. For your baby, having a sibling in the room can provide reassurance, and may even limit nighttime wakefulness.

Does your baby still have a late-night feed before you go to bed? Most babies drop this feed around the time they begin eating solids, but if you're still giving it, will feeding your baby late at night disturb her sibling? Do you have one late sleeper and one early riser? If so, how can you minimize the chances of early mornings for everyone?

Finally, if the sibling is a toddler, make sure that there are no small or otherwise dangerous objects around that she can pass through the bars of a cot. And check that your toddler can't somehow lift your baby out. Although you don't eradicate this eventuality if you give your children separate rooms (a mobile toddler can still go into the baby's room), the temptation is much greater if your baby is in the same space.

Sleep cycles

At birth, your baby may have slept for around 16 hours a day, perhaps even a bit more – with periods of sleep regularly interspersed with waking time to feed and, gradually, play. By six months old, your baby will be sleeping for around 13 to 14 hours a day, and by the time she reaches 12 months old, around 12 to 14 hours a day.

Sleep schedules

Your baby's longest sleep should be during the night now – a glorious 11 or so hours when everyone in the house is asleep. The remainder of her sleep time will occur during, usually, two daytime naps. You will probably have already established a bedtime routine, but if not now is the time to lay it down – you may find that once she passes the nine-month mark, she is too opinionated to be easily manipulated into doing things that work for you as a family.

There is advice on how to create a bedtime routine on pages 38–9. When you set the routine, make sure that it's workable for all of you. For example, if one of you comes home from work and wants to have time to play, perhaps bedtime needs to be a little later; or, find other times that you can dedicate as "fun time" with the parent who comes home later (see box, right).

Build in fun time at weekends if working hours mean you miss out during the week.

When your baby wakes in the morning, let her do this naturally (if you need her to wake at a certain time, turn on a light or open the curtains). Leave her in her cot to kick about a little, which encourages her to occupy herself if you need to get dressed before tending to her. See pages 66–7 for advice on babies who are early risers.

Daytime naps continue to be important elements in your baby's sleep routine.

As well as a long nighttime sleep, your baby will probably nap twice a day: once in the morning and once early afternoon. Some babies have a shorter morning nap, say 30 minutes or so around 9.30am, and a longer afternoon nap of an hour and a half; while others take two equal length naps. Think too about what works best for you, especially if you have other children. A baby who has a long afternoon nap may sleep through the moment you need to leave for the school run – in which case two equal naps may be better, or an afternoon nap that begins at 1pm rather than 1.30pm.

By six months old, most babies won't need an early evening nap. In fact, allowing one may interfere with nighttime sleep. Instead, if your baby seems to be struggling by the end of the day, engage her in an activity that's calming, but won't send her to sleep. Singing songs or reading books with sounds are good options. If you have other children, suggest everyone has some downtime as evening approaches. School-age siblings may even be the ones to read the stories. Your baby will love it!

"I'm home!" – the returning parent

It can be hard for the person who is out all day to walk through the door to find their baby bathed and almost ready for bed. Agree between you how you can ensure that you both have lots of opportunity to bond with your baby without disrupting her bedtime routine. Earmark parts of the routine that can be handed over to the returning parent when he or she is back in time. Keep the content of the routine the same each night: it can be helpful for your baby to learn that either one of you can take over. Here are some ways in which a working parent can feel involved:

- **Try baby massage**. This wonderful bonding activity has a calming influence that makes it perfect for a bedtime routine. You can massage through her sleepsuit if she's ready for bed.
- **Read your baby** a bedtime story, or sing a bedtime song.
- **Earmark time** on non-working days for your baby and the more absent parent to have fun together. Encourage this! It means you get time to indulge yourself, or to spend quality time with your other children. Hand over the whole bedtime routine on those days, too.

Separation anxiety

Between six and 12 months old, your baby will be on the move. With this growing independence comes an increasing sense that she's separate from you, a realization that comes with some inevitable hiccups. One of these is that at some point she may object to being left alone to sleep, both at naptimes and during the night. Although this apparent step backwards can be frustrating, treat it as a reassuring sign that she's developing in all the right ways. The quicker your baby understands that you will always come back to her, the quicker she will overcome separation anxiety. Try the following strategies to help her learn that she can rely upon you to reappear.

A dawning sense that she's separate from you can create a

Play peekaboo

This age-old game provides an early teaching tool for the notion that you can go and come back. Hide behind your hands or a muslin square. Disappear and pop out quickly at first, then as your baby gets used to the game, wait a few moments before reappearing. Let your baby have a turn – she can disappear too! Once she's more mobile, try hide and seek instead.

Clatter about in another room

If you have a safe place to leave your baby, such as in a cot or with someone you trust, pop out of the room and make some noise out of sight. She may object to you leaving at first, but if she can hear you nearby and then you return after a minute or two, she'll get used to the fact that she doesn't need to see you to know you're there. If she yells in objection, call back "I'm coming!" before you rush back in. She knows your voice, so will be reassured to hear it even if she can't see you.

feeling of vulnerability.

Don't vanish

Don't sneak away while your baby's back is turned. Be confident and smiley about leaving: say a firm good-bye and return when you say you will. Use positive communication and body language. If you aren't worried about leaving her, she'll learn not to worry, too.

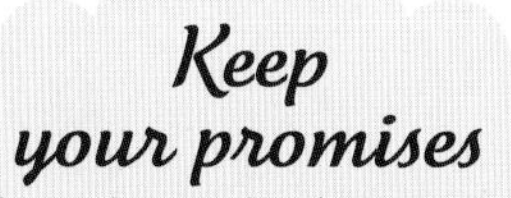

Keep your promises

Your baby understands what you say to her long before she can talk. If you're about to leave a room, tell her you're going, but that you'll be back soon, and return within one or two minutes. Keep other promises, too. If you tell her you'll take her to the swings later, do this. In these ways you'll earn her trust.

Bedtime reassurances

Here are a few additional strategies to put in place for bedtime.

Stick to your bedtime routine. Even if your baby's objections begin as soon as she has the first bedtime cue, follow the routine as normal. Bear in mind that in the end routine provides a sense of security for your baby. You can add a positive "Night, night! See you soon" if it helps – but remember to keep your promise and go back "soon" to check on her. When you leave the room again, perhaps say "See you in the morning!". And if she continues to cry, rather than rushing back in, call out to let her know you're close by.

If you can, try letting someone else do bedtime a couple of nights a week, so that your baby learns to feel safe in the care of others. If you aren't breastfeeding, get your partner, or someone else close to your baby, to give the last bottle of the night; and if you are breastfeeding, consider expressing that last feed so that someone else can give it.

Separation crying can be very distressing, but remember that your baby needs to learn from you that there is nothing to be worried about. If you do have to go back to her, don't do so in an anxious manner or obviously upset – try to keep your demeanour calm, confident, and positive.

Return to night wakings

Just when you think you've got your baby sleeping through until morning, she starts to wake up crying two, or even three, times a night. What has changed?

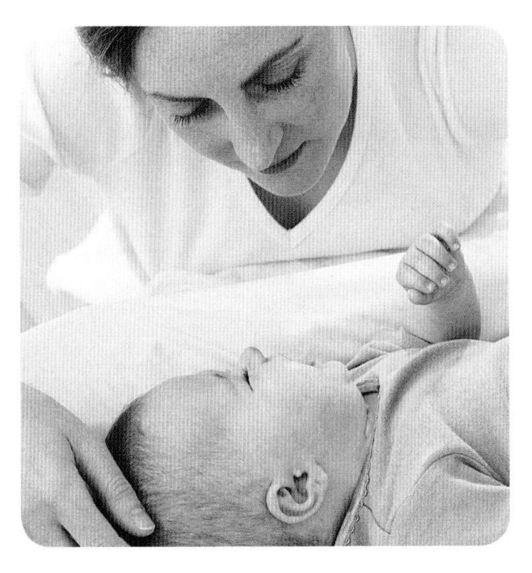

Separation anxiety

Probably the most likely explanation for a sudden return to nighttime waking is that your baby is starting to develop a sense of herself. When she wakes in the night and remembers that you aren't there, her instinct is to call out so that you come. See pages 50–1 for tips and techniques on how to cope with this phase.

New skills

This is a time of rapid learning for your baby, when she is processing and making sense of all her new skills. If she wakes in the night, she might like to try them out, or let you know about them there and then.

If she has just learned to crawl, for example, she may decide that the middle of the night is a good time to practise, even in her cot; and if she has learned to pull herself up to standing, she could get stuck up there – lots of babies learn to pull up before they learn to bend their knees to sit down again! Her only option, therefore, is to shout for help.

Develop a consistent system for putting her back to sleep when she calls. Try not to pick her up, talk to, or engage with her. Simply lie her back down or reposition her, give her a soothing pat, and leave the room. If she calls out again, go back and repeat the ritual of lying her down without making eye contact or talking. If she thinks there's no fun to be had by calling you to see how clever she is, she'll soon save her performance for when you're more interested.

Weaning

If you've just begun weaning your baby (see p54), the changes in her digestion may be keeping her awake – rather like how an adult might find it hard to sleep after a heavy meal. In the early stages of weaning, give her main "meal" at lunchtime, leaving plenty of time for digestion before bed. Once she is eating three meals a day, if practical, make teatime the lightest of the three, and give it at least two hours before bed. If at six months you haven't yet started weaning, consider whether nighttime waking might be because she's hungry.

Environmental triggers

Your baby likes consistency. Has something changed in her routine or environment that might be causing nighttime waking? It's perfectly normal for babies to take time to settle into a room of their own, for example – see pages 46–7 for tips on how best to make this transition. Even coming back to her own room after a holiday or weekend at Grandma's can have an unsettling effect.

Or has there been a change in the weather? Consider whether it might be too warm or too cold in her room and take away or add blankets as necessary. Our body temperature reaches its lowest at around three in the morning, so if this is roughly the time your baby is waking, being too cold may very well be the cause of her disrupted sleep.

Growth spurt

Babies have a growth spurt at both six months and again at nine months old. Although they last only a few days, growth spurts can cause increased nighttime wakefulness (although conversely they may instead make your baby sleep better than usual). See pages 42–3 for more information.

Teething

It's likely that somewhere around the six-month-old mark (sometimes earlier and sometimes later), your baby's first teeth will start to come through. Even long before these appear, her gums may ache and become sore, causing her to wake at night. Other signs of teething include increased dribbling, flushed cheeks, a runny nose, and an increased need to gnaw, and she may even be off her food. If you think this might be the problem, you can try to relieve her discomfort at night by rubbing a clean finger over her gum, or, if she seems to be in a lot of discomfort, try a little teething gel or the correct dosage of infant paracetamol or ibuprofen. Consult your health visitor if this continues to disrupt her sleep.

Sore, niggly gums can disturb your older baby's sleep.

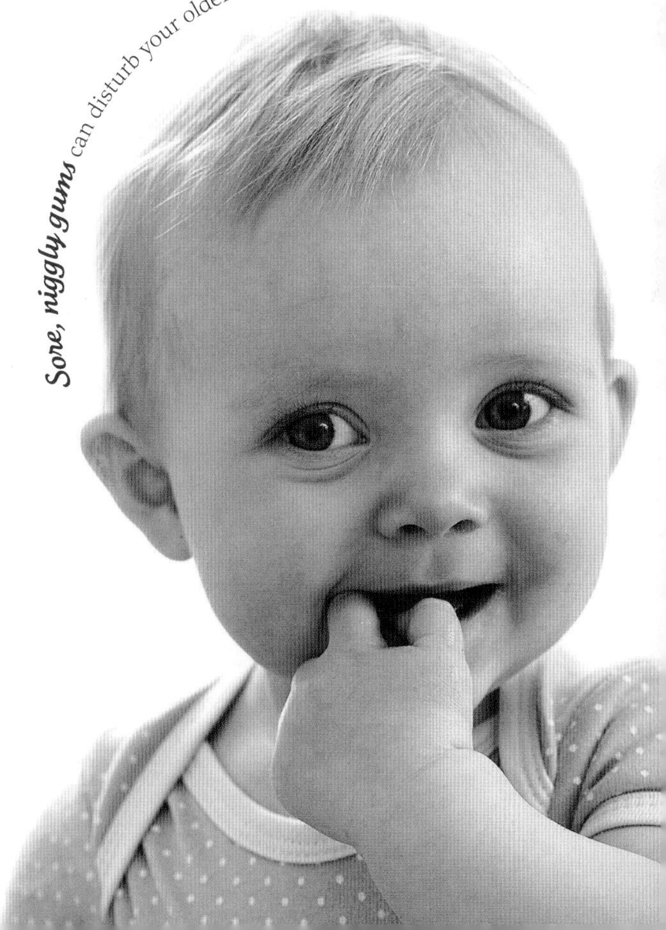

Feeding at night

In a perfect world, by the time your baby reaches six months old, she would happily be having all her feeds during the day and sleeping through the night uninterrupted. However, some babies need a little bit more encouragement than others to drop their nighttime feed.

Just for comfort?

One reason why feeding at night can become a habit is that it's a source of comfort for your little one. If you think this is the case, make sure she has plenty of loving attention in the day, and a soothing bedtime routine so she goes to bed feeling happy and content.

Why nighttime feeds may still happen

There are two main reasons why, at six months old, your baby might still wake during the night for a feed. The first is that she isn't getting enough calories during the day to sustain her; and the second is that waking for a feed at night has become a habit rather than a necessity.

Starting weaning

Guidelines suggest that at around six months your baby's digestive system is developed enough to cope with solid foods. Moreover, while milk continues to be her main source of nutrition for a while, her body now needs other foods to provide the range of nutrients needed for growth and development. In particular, by six months, the iron in breast milk is no longer sufficient to meet your baby's energy needs.

Waking for a feed in the night can be a sign she is ready for solids. Other signs include showing an interest in your food, continuing to be restless still after a good milk feed, or gnawing on her hands. She may not have gained weight despite being well, and if she can hold her neck unsupported, she's physically ready to learn to swallow. Gentle weaning onto baby porridge or single-vegetable purées mixed with breast milk or formula, given a teaspoon at a time in the day, can provide sustenance to last the night.

If she continues to wake for a night feed after starting weaning, this is probably because doing so has become habitual.

Babies who graze

Studies show that babies who are demand fed have a tendency to become grazers, feeding little and often, including into the night. If you think this is the case, start to reverse the process. Try to make sure that your baby takes full, regular milk feeds in the day. At six months she should be able to go four hours without needing a snack. Once she can achieve this, she's ready to break her nighttime habit.

Breaking the habit

The steps below can help you break the habit of nighttime feeds in your older baby.

Resist the temptation to let your baby fall asleep while she is feeding (see p39).
While this can make for an easier transition from your arms back into her cot, she may well come to depend on this to help her fall asleep. She is also less likely to take a full feed if she falls asleep during it.

Gradually reduce the quantity of milk during night feeds.
On each consecutive night give 25ml/1fl oz less milk than the night before; or, if you're breastfeeding, reduce the time your baby feeds by around two to three minutes each night. Remember, too, to interact with your baby as little as possible during these nighttime feeds – it may, after all, not be the food she's looking for, but your attention. The process needs to be gradual. It may take up to two weeks to completely wean your baby off her nighttime feed, but hopefully by the end of that time, if she does still wake, you'll be able to settle her back to sleep with a gentle pat of reassurance, and then as long as she's eating enough during the day, she'll sleep through without waking at all.

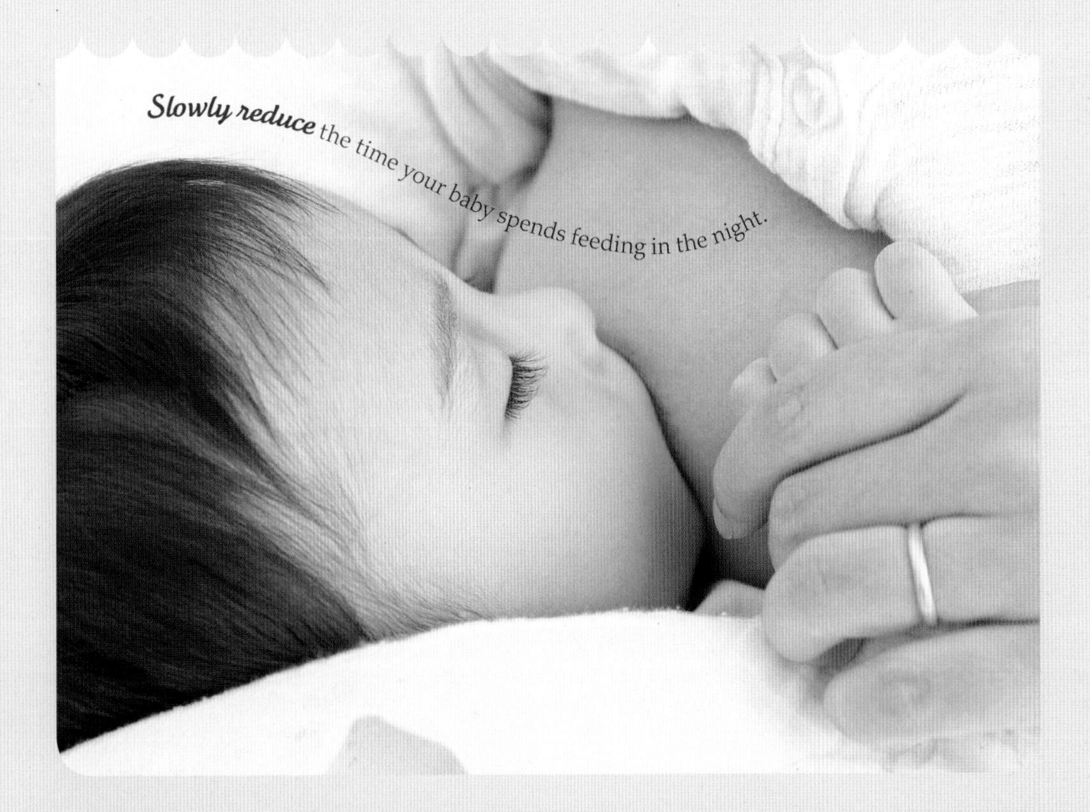
Slowly reduce the time your baby spends feeding in the night.

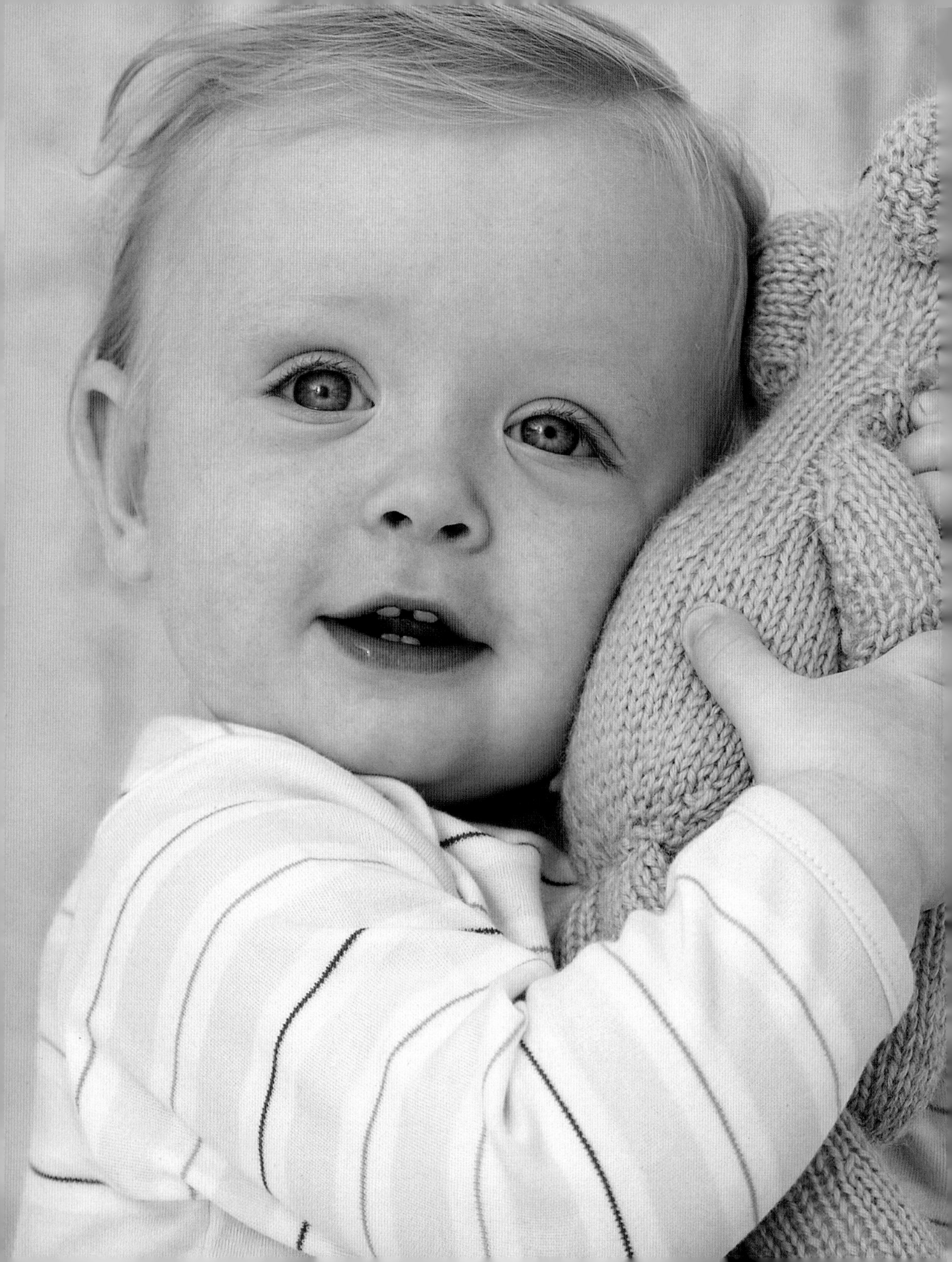

5

12 to 18 months

Between 12 and 18 months old, many babies will become fully mobile. Bottom shuffling, crawling, or walking, this is a new age of independence for your developing child. With this independence comes a greater sense of self, which for your baby's sleep can mean problems with settling caused by ongoing "separation anxiety" as your baby becomes more aware of when you're not there; and you may also encounter a certain amount of bedtime wilfulness. In this chapter, we look at how to improve sleep quality for all of you as you move from having a young baby in the family to having an active toddler.

Sleeping spaces

Now that your baby can move around, his cot is no longer the safe place it might once have been. It may very quickly become a climbing frame and he may even be able to escape altogether! Of course, his new-found skills as an acrobat are not necessarily moderated by any sense of danger.

Cot safety

As soon as your baby can pull himself to standing (even if he can't walk yet), make sure that the cot base is on its lowest setting and, if relevant, the sides of the cot are lockable, or ideally fixed, in their uppermost position. Tighten any screws and make sure that any sliding mechanisms fit snugly into their runners – even if he doesn't try to launch himself over the side, your toddler could catch or pinch his fingers in the gaps. Make sure that there's nothing in the cot, such as big, stuffed toys, that could raise your toddler up so that he could reach his leg over the side.

Don't be complacent. Even if you think it looks highly unlikely that your toddler could reach over and topple out, be vigilant about this possibility and take steps to remove any danger – even, in some cases, considering an early transition to a child bed (see pp70–1). Bear in mind that some small children can perform quite remarkable feats of acrobatics! Make sure that if he does fall out, there are no sharp corners nearby for him to topple on to and hurt himself on, and perhaps even consider a soft rug as a landing mat just in case.

Keeping warm

Now that your toddler can move, even well-tucked-in sheets and blankets will provide little resistance against his attempts to wriggle free. This can mean that he wakes feeling cold in the night. A toddler sleeping bag that pops over the shoulders is a good way to overcome this, but bear in mind that it can cause your toddler to trip if he tries to stand up in it. A fleecy sleepsuit that has feet and legs and zips up the middle may be a better option.

Roaming free

Once your toddler gets to 18 months old, it's perfectly possible that he will be able to climb out of the cot safely and roam free. Consider how far you want him to be able to get during any nighttime or early morning adventures.

If he has been used to sleeping with the door closed, that may be enough to keep him contained within his bedroom, at least until he can reach or operate the door handle. Make sure there are no choking or trip hazards (such as window blind cords or electrical leads) that

Back to your bed

Make a decision now about a strategy if your toddler crawls into your bed at night. Will you let him in for a cuddle any time, or keep it as a morning or weekend-only treat? Remember, though, that all days are the same to him. Or perhaps you will put him straight back in his cot.

might be dangerous for him, and put safety plugs in any visible or reachable electric sockets. Ensure, too, that he can't climb up on anything, such as a chair or low shelf, to reach a window.

As your baby's mobility increases, you will need to consider every scenario.

It is never safe to lock the door to your baby's room to prevent him from getting out – you need to be able to get in there quickly, or him out quickly, in case of emergency. If he sleeps with the door open, think about whether you need to install a stair gate. Position it in the doorway to his room if you want to stop him getting any further; or at the top of the stairs if you want him to be able to find you, but keep him safe from any tumbles.

Consider the sleep of any other children in your household when you make your decision – perhaps your toddler would be more likely to wake an older sibling to play than to come to find you? What impact would that have on your other children's sleep?

If your toddler does consistently wander into a sibling's room during the night, and perhaps even tries to curl up with them to sleep, you might want to consider whether it might be better for everyone to let them share a room if there is space – and with the sibling's permission, of course.

Sleep cycles

Between the ages of 12 and 18 months old, your baby's body clock should come more into line with your own. The fact that you've established bright mornings, regular mealtimes, consistent nap- and bedtimes, and darkness at night is starting to pay off.

How much sleep?

At a year old, toddlers still need around 12 to 14 hours nighttime sleep and around two hours of napping in every 24-hour period, but by the time your baby reaches 18 months old (usually between the 16- and 18-month mark), he may need only one longer nap (of say two hours), most likely taken in the afternoon. He may still need a quiet wind-down period at some other point in the day, though.

A time of transition

Adjusting to fewer daytime naps can be tough for parents. When will you catch up on paperwork, chores, or your own rest? The plus side is that you and your toddler are freed up more in the day, and coping without a morning nap will help him prepare for preschool playgroups.

Dropping a nap

The biggest tell-tale sign that your toddler is ready to drop his morning nap is that you put him in his cot as usual, but find that he spends the time simply playing in there, or calling for you and trying to climb out, rather than actually sleeping. He may even refuse to get into his cot at all!

However, the transition between two daytime naps and one can be tricky for both parents and babies. Your newly established routine may seem to work on one day, but then fall by the wayside the next, simply because your baby isn't quite ready to cope every day without a morning nap.

To help ease the way, tune in to your toddler's sleepy signs. If, just as you ready the buggy for a morning activity, he seems cranky or tearful, or is a little detached, rubbing his eyes or yawning, this could in fact be a day for a morning nap. If he gets to almost lunchtime and then starts showing his sleepy signs, consider giving him his lunch a little early and then putting him to bed for his afternoon nap a little early, too.

You'll probably find that, on the days when he doesn't have his morning nap, he'll sleep longer during his afternoon nap for a few weeks. Try to schedule the nap with an earlier start time rather than letting him sleep late into the afternoon. As long as he is waking from his afternoon nap at his usual time, he should still be able to settle down at night.

Accept that daytime routines may be thrown while your toddler adjusts to his new sleep schedule.

Nonetheless, with only one nap notched up during the day, you may find that initially your toddler seems ready for bedtime earlier than usual. Stick as closely as you can to the routine you've already established, but perhaps extend your baby's quiet time before bed, or have a slightly longer bath. The key is to try to keep your toddler's body clock set to the same nighttime sleep and morning waking schedules, and to make allowances for changes in routine during the time inbetween.

New baby on the way

Dealing with pregnancy and with a toddler is almost as demanding as dealing with a new baby and a toddler, and it could feel like the last thing you need is for your toddler to drop one of his naps. During the time when he would once have had a morning nap, have some quiet time together, reading or doing puzzles. Some mothers have a small toy box filled with special toys that come out only when mummy is resting. The idea is that these toys – which aren't always available – hold your toddler's attention a little longer, giving you some time to rest. Another good idea is to get out the photo albums of your toddler as a baby. Children love to look at themselves in photos and hear stories about their babyhood, and it's a wonderful way to cuddle up together and introduce the idea of having a tiny baby in the house.

Remember that, for you, resting is almost as restorative as sleeping itself, and down time will give you both an opportunity to keep up your energy levels for the more active parts of the day. Then, when your toddler is sleeping during the afternoon, take the opportunity to have a snooze. Set your alarm if you're worried that you won't wake up when you need to.

Bedtime resistance

Along with all the developmental leaps your baby has made in his first year comes the ability to think more independently and to make some decisions of his own. You might see this at mealtimes if he refuses certain foods, or when he resists you trying to strap him into his buggy. It's also perfectly normal for this newfound confidence to manifest itself at bedtime.

Finding ways to resist

There are three main ways in which your toddler may try to resist going to bed. The first is outright refusal. He may simply pretend he hasn't heard you, or perhaps he makes loud and stubborn protestations: "No!". Alternatively, or additionally, he may get out of bed once you are out of the room. And finally, he may use delay tactics. If your toddler is asking for one more game in the bath, one more song, one more bedtime story, or one more cuddle, he's probably trying to keep you going to stave off the inevitable.

Overcoming resistance

Once he's over a year old, your toddler will probably want to have some control over his life. One way in which he can exercise that

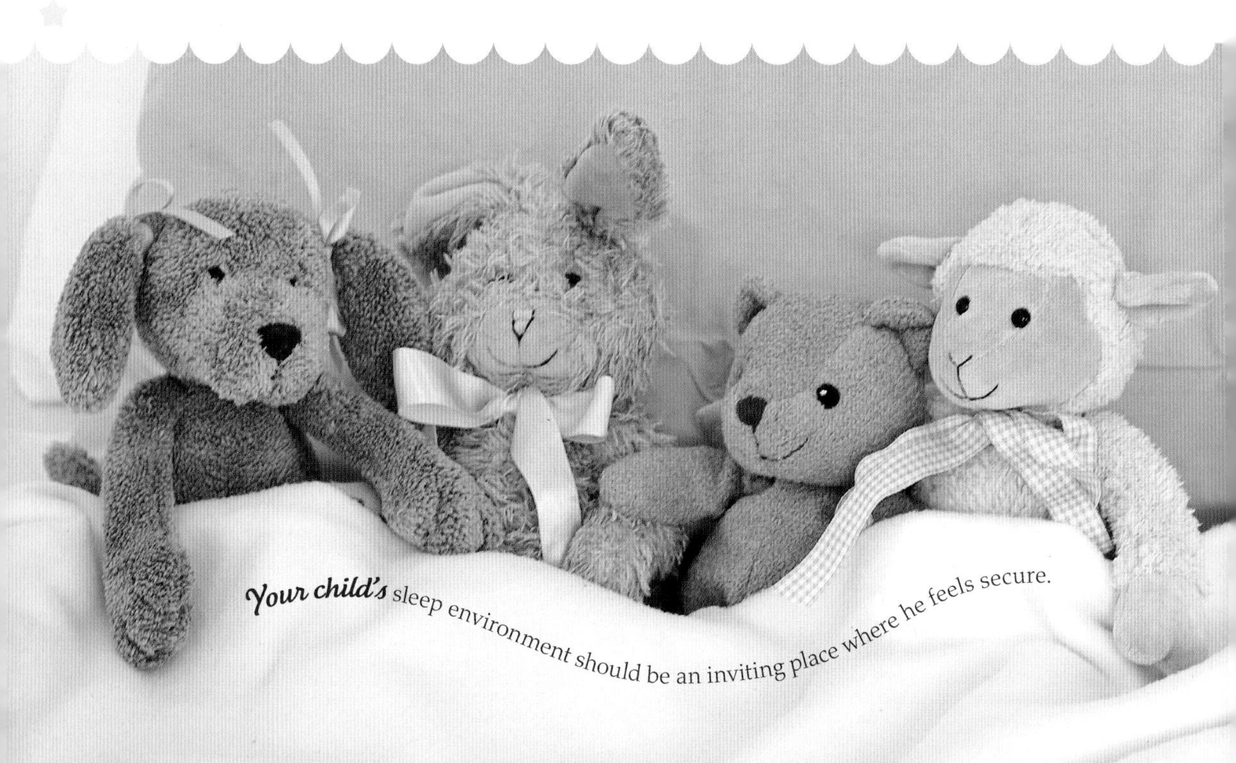

Your child's sleep environment should be an inviting place where he feels secure.

Happy associations

It's important that your toddler makes only happy associations with his bedroom. Fill it with images that make him happy, such as photographs of family, as well as with favourite toys, and paint it a calming colour. Avoid using it as a place of punishment.

control is to show you that he knows he has a choice – and he's not going to choose what you want him to do. Try letting him feel that he has more of a say in his bedtime routine. Give him simple choices about the peripheral matters of going to bed. For example, perhaps you could ask him which teddies he wants to say goodnight to and lay them out ready for him before he has his bath. You could offer him a choice of the green or the blue towel when he comes out of the bath, or to have bubbles or not to have bubbles; and let him decide which pyjamas he would like to wear tonight. If there are many options for the pyjamas, offer a choice of two to limit the opportunity for conflict. Hopefully, he will be so distracted by being such a master of his own destiny, the act of actually getting into his cot and settling down to sleep will seem simply the natural conclusion to all the important decisions he has just made.

If he still tries to delay bedtime, you need to set the boundaries and stick to them. Perhaps he has always had one story, one song, one game in the bath – in which case be very clear that that's the way it's going to stay, and make sure that anyone else who puts him to bed sticks to this, too. Avoid the temptation to have "special nights" when it's okay to have one more story – bear in mind that your toddler has no concept that one day is different from another. If he protests that he's not tired, that's fine, but make it clear that you are still not going to change bedtime. Instead, kindly let him know that, even if he lies awake, bedtime is now. Try not to let it become a battle of wills, though. If you are consistent and kind, but firm, after a week or so of realizing that his attempts at prolonging bedtime aren't getting him anywhere, he's likely to give up.

Make your toddler's room a comfortable and inviting place to give him one less reason to resist bedtime.

If he has a bed (see pp70–1) and regularly gets out of it, you'll need resilience and patience, but the solution is often simple. Take him back into his room without engaging with him – no eye contact or talking – and gently put him back to bed. If he refuses to lie down, don't enter into a discussion, just leave the room. Repeat this for as many times as he tries to escape. He'll most likely lose interest eventually.

Habitual waking

There are many reasons why toddlers can form a habit of night waking. It can be a hangover from waking for a feed, or your little one may have had a period of anxiety, illness, or disruption, and although the trigger has gone, he has got used to waking and calling for you. If he had a spate of nightmares, he may still wake for reassurance. Whatever the cause, putting in place strategies during the day and night can help him kick the habit.

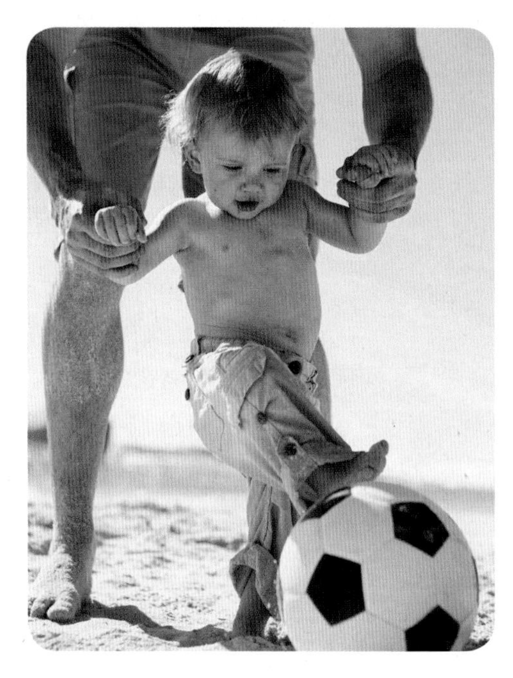

Good tiredness

Make sure your toddler is properly tired by the end of the day. Fill his days with activity, while still observing naptimes (an overtired toddler will be too wired to sleep, so naps are important). Play in the garden or park, go swimming, or do puzzles or painting. Then follow your bedtime routine, and hope that the busy day will help him sleep more soundly.

Daytime fluids

Some toddlers wake because they think they are thirsty. Try to make sure that your child has plenty of water or diluted fresh juice (dilute juice 50:50 with water) throughout the day. Aim to give six to eight small cups of "good" fluids daily. Avoid squash and fizzy drinks, and avoid juice after 3pm – sugary drinks will give him an energy boost that he doesn't need before bedtime. If he wakes in the night asking for water, unless it is very hot or he could be dehydrated owing to illness, try to resist, simply reassuring him back to sleep.

Occupy your little one in the day with both physical and mental activities.

If you have the opposite problem and your toddler drinks too much fluid towards the end of the day, resulting in a sodden nappy in the middle of the night, try to make sure he has most of his fluids before lunchtime, and then offer just a small cup of water mid-afternoon and with his tea, before his bedtime milk. Don't restrict fluids, just change when you give them.

Nighttime strategies

Habitual waking is waking without a real need, but at more or less the same time every night. If a few nights of simply lying your baby back down doesn't break the habit, try this more radical strategy, often used to overcome habitual wakings or nightmares in adults. Set your alarm and gently wake your baby shortly before the time of his habitual waking. Try not to rouse him fully, just disturb him enough to make him stir, then pat and soothe him so he goes back to sleep. The idea is that you will have interrupted the sleep cycle (see p36) from which he usually wakes up. When he falls back to sleep after you've roused him, he will begin a new sleep cycle and the hope is that he won't come fully into consciousness in the gap between subsequent cycles. After a few successful nights using this strategy, try leaving him all night – hopefully you will have done enough to break the habit altogether.

Give plenty of fluids during the day.

Moving home

Significant life events, such as moving home, can cause something called Adjustment Sleep Disorder in children, which is when the period of adjustment to a new situation or scenario causes a return to a previous nighttime waking habit.

Be patient and consistent in your approach as you try to correct this, starting with a return to the basics. Make sure your baby has plenty of familiar things around him in his new room – the same pictures on the wall, the same toys to play with, and the same cot and bedding. Follow your bedtime routine just as you did before – it's more important than ever that your baby experiences consistency. When you put him down to bed, make sure he is drowsy, but that he hasn't fallen asleep in your arms – he has to be aware of where he's going to bed, so that he's not confused if he wakes during the night. If he does wake in the night, follow the same strategies that you had in place for dealing with night waking in your old home, but start at the beginning again. So, for example, if you settled him by going in at increasing intervals (see pp90–1), begin that process again so that you re-build his confidence that all is well.

Early rising

Just when you think you've cracked your baby's nighttime waking, early morning waking takes its place.

Nature or nurture?

You'll know simply from the people you've met during your life that some like to get up with the lark while others would rather sleep until a hurricane forces them from their slumber. The same is true for babies – except that both personalities may go through a phase of waking up too early. So, do you have a natural lark, or is it just that your toddler is waking too early during his final sleep cycle?

Your toddler's morning behaviour will tell you. If he wakes up at 5am, singing and chatting brightly, ready to play, and showing no signs of needing a nap until after lunch, he is a lark. On the other hand, if he wakes and is then cranky and tired all morning, then it's likely he needed more sleep, but for some reason didn't get it.

The following strategies, see right, are intended to solve the latter problem. You can try them with your lark and they may work, but don't necessarily expect success. Instead, in a lark's case, consider pushing back his bedtime so that he starts his sleep later, then wakes later in the morning (do this gradually over the course of one or two weeks, making bedtime 10 minutes later at a time). At the same time, encourage him to occupy himself in his cot when he wakes. Hand him a toy to play with and let him know that mummy will be back when it's time to get up.

Playing a game at the crack of

Encourage self-settling

Your baby's early waking may simply be an habitual waking happening in the early morning rather than in the night. When he wakes like this in the night, you would simply settle him down, but as it's light, you think he has woken for the day. Try one of the strategies on pages 86–93 to help overcome this, and ensure that he goes to bed sleepy, but not asleep, so that he can learn to settle himself back to sleep if he wakes.

dawn may be fun for your baby, but wearing for you!

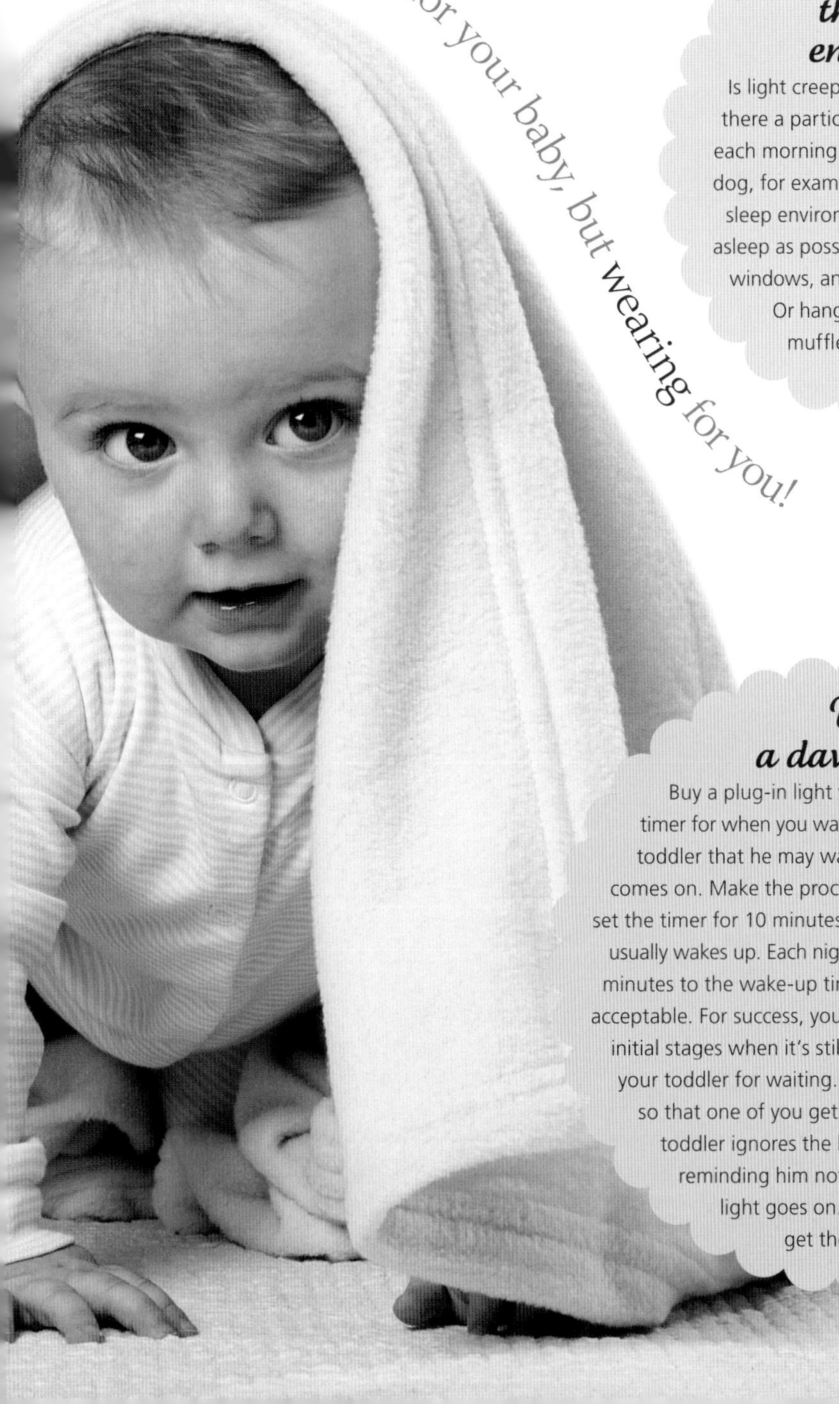

Check the sleeping environment

Is light creeping in around the curtains? Is there a particular street noise that happens each morning at his waking hour – a barking dog, for example? Do all you can to make his sleep environment as conducive to staying asleep as possible. Put blackout blinds on the windows, and consider secondary glazing. Or hang heavy fabric curtains to muffle noise as well as block out the light.

Use a dawn light

Buy a plug-in light with a timer, setting the timer for when you want to get up. Explain to your toddler that he may wake you only when the light comes on. Make the process gradual. On the first night, set the timer for 10 minutes later than the time your toddler usually wakes up. Each night (or every two nights), add 10 minutes to the wake-up time until you reach a time that's acceptable. For success, you will need to get up (even in the initial stages when it's still too early for you), and praise your toddler for waiting. Take turns with your partner, so that one of you gets a full night's sleep. If your toddler ignores the light, lie him back down, reminding him not to wake you until the light goes on. Eventually he will get the message.

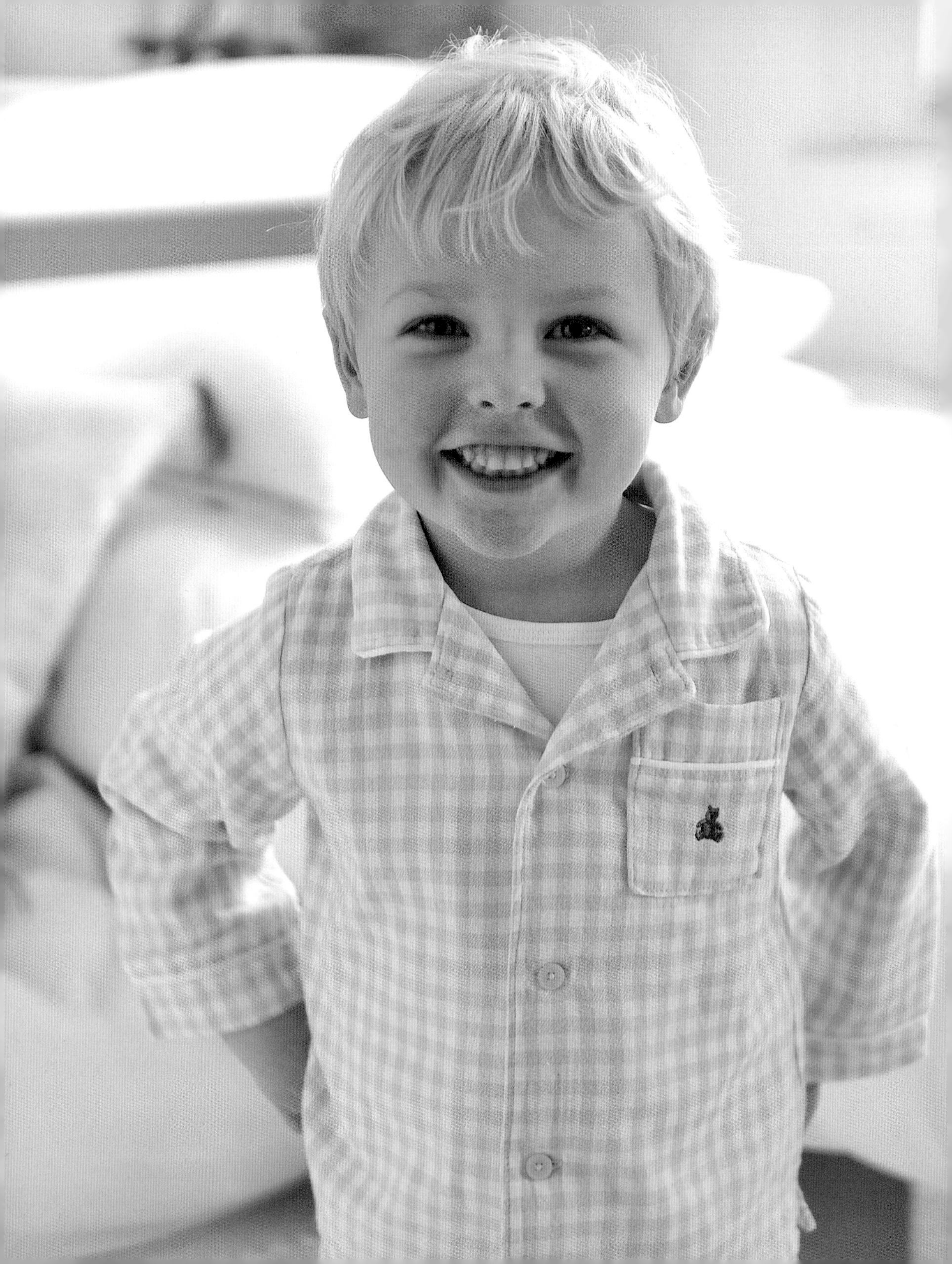

6

18 months to 3 years

It probably seems a long time ago that your baby was waking every few hours in the night to feed. Since those early weeks, you have managed to teach him the difference between night and day, you have set his body clock to fall into line with your own, and you have taught him to become a more independent, confident individual. Now is the time to consolidate the work you've done, reinforcing all the good sleep habits you've established. In this chapter, you'll learn how your toddler's sleep finally comes closer to the patterns of adult sleep, as well as how to ease the transition to a "big bed", and deal with issues such as nightmares.

Where your toddler sleeps

At some time around the age of two years old, children are usually ready to move into a "big bed". This time can be both exciting and unsettling for your toddler as she leaves the safe confines of her cot.

Not quite ready

If you've moved your toddler to a bed, but she finds it hard to settle, refuses to get in, or gets up and wanders around, have you made the transition too early? Try for two weeks to get her used to her bed, but if things don't improve, reinstate her cot, without making this seem a punishment.

Deciding when to make the move

Has your toddler grown too large for her cot? When she stands up in it, does the side of the cot come up to mid-chest height? If so, she is probably tall enough to climb out if she tried and could potentially harm herself.

Not having enough width to roll comfortably, or bumping her head against the top of the cot are also signs she has grown out of it.

If your toddler is a second or subsequent child, or if she has friends who have made the transition, she may ask to move out of her cot in a desire to be like other children. Capitalize on her positive attitude and take the plunge while she is willing to embrace this change.

Finally, avoid switching to a big bed during times of other change – if you're potty training, for example. Do one thing at a time.

Moving to a big bed is a childhood rite of passage – a step towards independence.

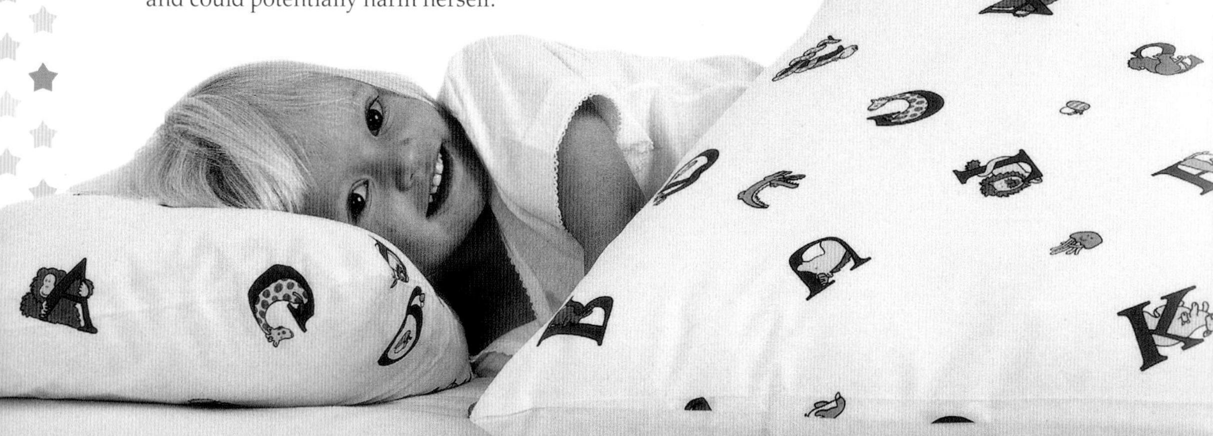

Choosing the right bed

The time has come to make the transition, but what bed will you choose for your toddler? You might decide to start with a dedicated toddler bed or go straight to a full-size single bed. Toddler beds are low to the ground and tend to have an inbuilt guard-rail to stop your little one toppling out. You may also be able to use your cot mattress (which is both comforting to your toddler and a cost-saving for you), and all the same bedding. However, you will still need to replace the toddler bed with a full-size bed when your little one reaches about five years old. In which case, you may take the long view and go for a single bed straight away. If you do this, attach a guard-rail on any open sides to minimize the risk of your toddler rolling out and hurting or upsetting herself.

Easing the transition

Moving to a bed does not mean that any aspect of the bedtime routine should change, except perhaps that you can snuggle up together on the bed to read the bedtime story. If you can, position the bed exactly as you had the cot. Try to make sure that there is a wall at the head of the bed and a wall along one side.

Take your toddler shopping with you to choose the bed, or the bedding if you are not buying the bed itself new. Being able to choose a new cover, a pillow and pillowcase, or a blanket decorated with a favourite character will help your toddler feel that she has some control over the change and she'll be more likely to accept her new sleeping quarters.

Transfer any of your toddler's favourite toys or blankets to the new bed. Even if these blankets are too small now, they will be comfortingly familiar.

Safe sleeping

Avoid putting the bed next to a radiator (your toddler could scald herself if the radiator comes on), and near any loose cords or wires that she could tangle herself up in. Consider, too, how to keep your toddler safe if she gets out of bed and goes wandering (see p73).

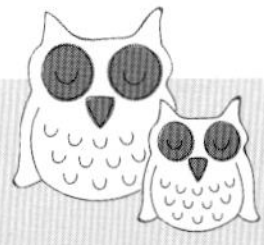

New bed, new baby

The impending arrival of a baby is another reason you may need to move your toddler to a big bed, to free up the cot – but take care to do this without your toddler feeling displaced.

As long as your toddler is older than 18 months, move her to a bed at least two months before the expected arrival of the baby. If you can, dismantle the cot and store it out of sight. Consider using new bedding for your baby: your toddler is more likely to remember patterns on a favourite blanket than the cot itself.

If your toddler is still too little to move out of her cot as the birth approaches, wait until your baby is about two months old and move your toddler then. By that time, your toddler will have had time to bond with the baby, and you may still have time for the cot to go out of sight before your baby actually needs it.

Staying in bed

Once you've moved your toddler from a cot into a bed – and if you have a climber, perhaps even before you make this move – you've opened the possibility for getting out of bed at will.

Setting the ground rules

Follow your bedtime routine as normal, but also work out how you will impress upon your toddler that once she is in bed she must stay there. If your toddler has never tried to crawl out of her cot, you might think that it's better not to draw attention to the fact that it's possible to get in and out of bed – many toddlers just stay in bed because that's what they've been used to doing.

An established bedtime routine should help your child continue to respond to the cues for sleeptime.

If, on the other hand, you think you might have a wanderer on your hands, consider all the possible excuses she might find to get out of bed, such as forgetting to brush her teeth, wanting a drink, needing to use the potty, or saying goodnight to Daddy or to a favourite teddy. Make a list and then every night check everything off it. Tell her how brilliant you think teddy is because he wants to snuggle down without moving the whole night. Tuck in your toddler and say goodnight in the usual way, then leave the room – the aim is that you give her no excuses to get up.

Have you tried?

Reward charts. Children thrive on reward and by the age of two, your toddler will get the concept. For each night she goes to bed happily and stays in bed, in the morning reward her with a star, or let her colour in a box on a chart. When her chart is filled, she gets a treat, such as a comic or fun activity.

Getting back into bed

If she does get out, tell her kindly, but firmly, that she must stay in bed, then take her back without saying anything more and with little interaction. Pop her back into bed, tuck her up, say goodnight (make it functional rather than lingering), and leave the room. You can use this tactic for nighttime creeping into your bed, too – make sure your partner is fully on board with the strategy, so that neither side of the bed becomes an okay place to sleep!

You will need patience and stamina as you may have to repeat this routine several times an evening for several nights, until she decides that getting out of bed is so boring that she opts to stay put. Be kind, firm, and consistent.

Using a barrier

If you find that taking your child back to bed isn't working – bearing in mind that it may take a few nights, or even a week or two of repetition for the message to sink in – you may consider using a barrier to prevent her from leaving her room. A stair gate across the doorway will enable you to leave the door open so that you can hear her, but keep her contained. However, a child who can climb over a cot could probably manage a stair gate too. You might decide to shut the door (never lock it for safety reasons) – you could use a low-wattage nightlight in the room if your toddler worries about the dark, and use a baby monitor if you're worried that you won't hear her. Don't use the barrier as punishment, for example, "If you don't stay in your bed, I will have to shut the door", as that will only build up negative associations with being in her room.

In the morning

Praise, praise, praise! Tell your little one how proud you were of her when she fell asleep in her big bed and how brilliant she was when she stayed in it. Avoid focusing on any negatives, for example, don't mention any repeated wanderings; it's better to pay those no attention at all.

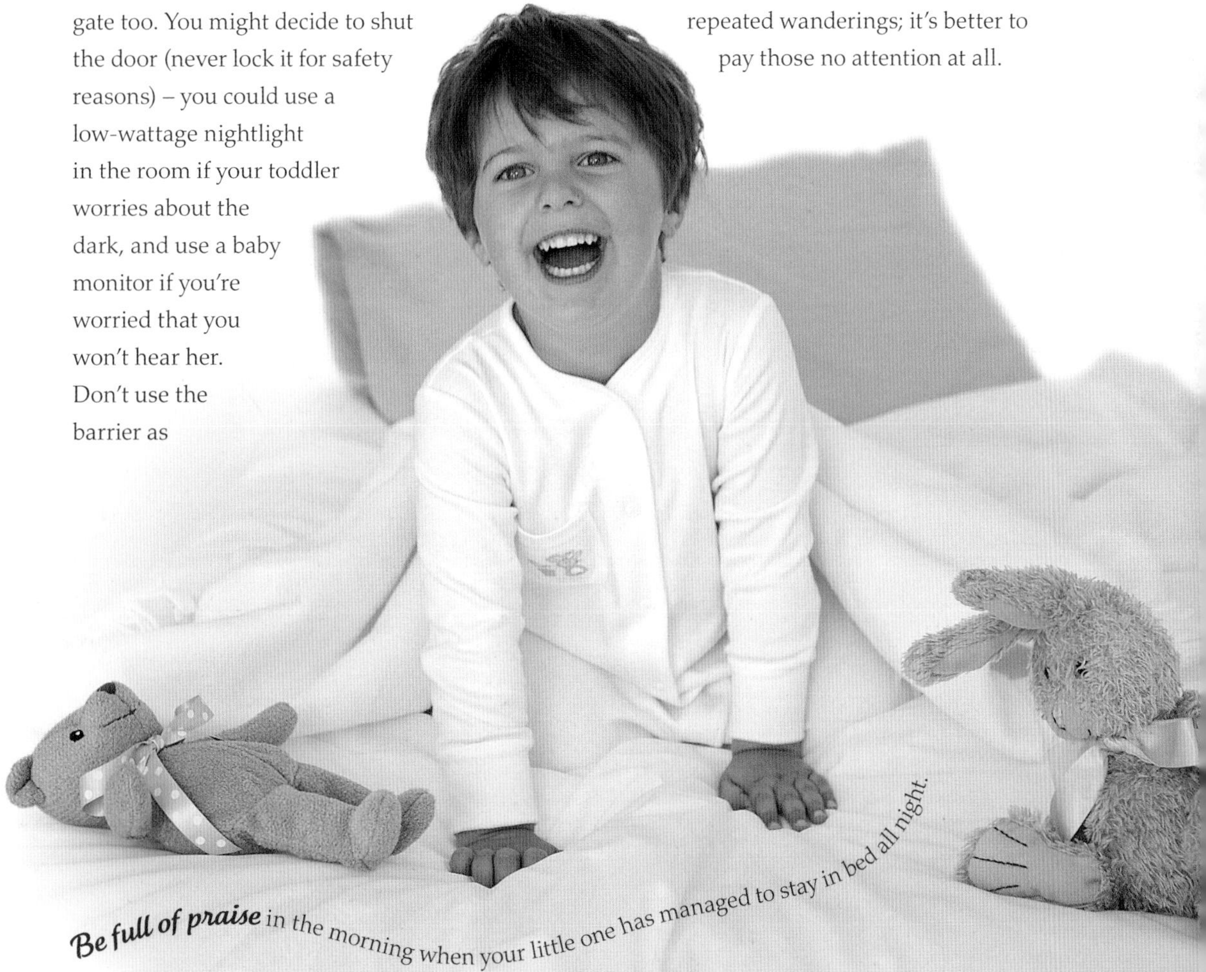

Be full of praise in the morning when your little one has managed to stay in bed all night.

Sleep cycles

In the preschool years, your toddler's sleep cycles edge closer to those of an adult (see p11). She still has cycles of about 60 minutes, but spends more time in deep sleep and less in light and dreaming sleep. By around the age of four, she has 90-minute cycles made up of all the stages of sleep: drowsy, light, deep, and dreaming. And, like you, she'll start the night mostly in deep sleep, with periods of light and dreaming sleep extending towards morning.

Dropping the afternoon nap

At some point between the ages of two and three years old, most toddlers will start to drop their afternoon nap, and by the age of four most will have dropped it completely. You will know your toddler is ready to leave her afternoon nap behind when she potters around in her bedroom rather than sleeping, or protests at being taken to bed in the afternoon at all. And you may find that on the days when she does sleep, she is less willing to go to bed in the evening, or wakes particularly early the next morning. Whatever the situation, don't let the afternoon nap become a time of contention, but do make sure that if napping isn't happening, quiet time (see top right) is.

On some days, the need for an afternoon nap will be apparent.

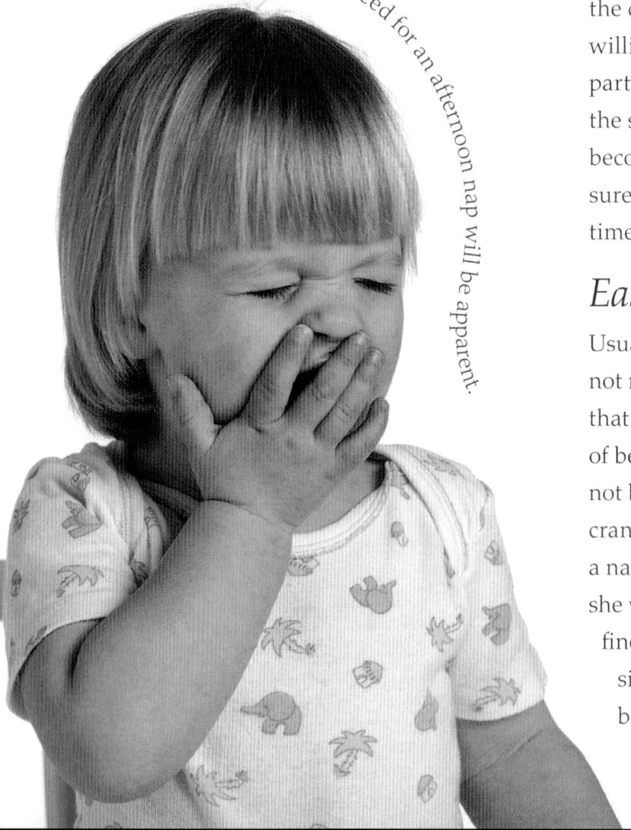

Easing the change

Usually, the transition between napping and not napping is a gradual one. You may find that on some days, your toddler shows signs of being tired – rubbing her eyes, yawning, not being able to concentrate, or getting cranky. On these days she probably still needs a nap if she's willing to settle. On other days, she will seem to be full of energy and clearly fine without her nap. Be prepared for up to six weeks of transition. Although life will be a little less predictable for a while, it's

Finding quiet time

On days when your toddler doesn't nap, have down time after lunch so you can both recharge and to ensure she isn't overtired at bedtime. Read a story or cuddle up and listen to an audio book. A little quiet TV is okay if she keeps still. Or encourage her to play quietly close by while you read or go online.

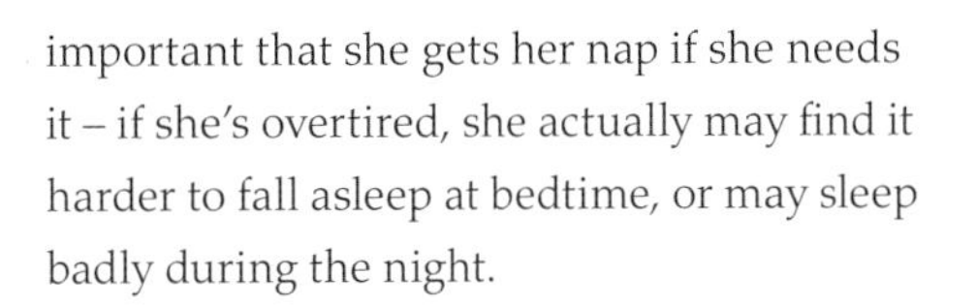

important that she gets her nap if she needs it – if she's overtired, she actually may find it harder to fall asleep at bedtime, or may sleep badly during the night.

Building flexibility into routines will help you cope with this time of transition.

You might find that in the early stages of transition, she will drop to sleep while in her buggy or car seat if you're out during the afternoon. That's fine, and it's probably better to let her have a snooze, but try not to let her snooze for too long or too late in the afternoon (say, not for longer than an hour and not later than 2.30pm).

If your toddler is struggling to make it through to bedtime on non-napping days, consider making bedtime 30 minutes earlier than usual for a while. Then, gradually, move her bedtime later again in five- or 10-minute increments until you are back to where you need to be. For example, if her bedtime used to be at 7pm, but in order to prevent her being overtired you move it back half an hour to 6.30pm, on subsequent nights add another five or 10 minutes to bedtime, to around 6.35 or 6.40pm and so on, until you are back at her regular 7pm bedtime.

Nappy-free nights

Although some toddlers will become nappy-free both day and night in one go, the process usually has two phases – toddlers will first learn to be dry during the day, but still wear a nappy at night, and then eventually (sometimes even a couple of years later) become dry at night, too. Take your toddler's lead and don't rush the process. Becoming dry at night requires hormonal changes that in some children take longer to happen than in others. If your toddler wakes in the morning with a dry nappy for five days in a row, give nappy-free nighttimes a go. If you find that she then starts to wake worried about going to the potty, or because she is wet, it could be too soon for this step. Without any fuss or recriminations, go back to nighttime nappies and save this second transition for another time.

Winding down (not up)

Young or old, for any of us to fall asleep easily, we need to be in a state of calm. With this in mind, it is generally unrealistic to expect an excited toddler to get into bed and fall fast asleep straight away.

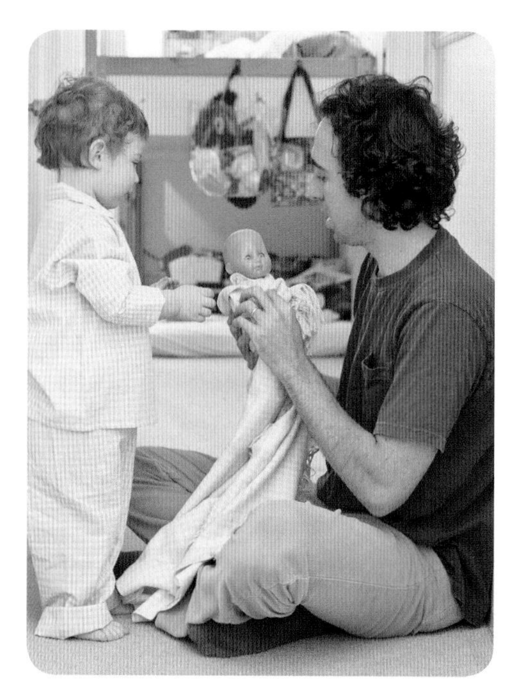

Quiet play

Although your toddler can't yet tell the time, she can attune to phases of the day. In the morning there is a bustle of activity as the day gathers pace. Then, perhaps there's time with friends or a toddler group before lunchtime. After lunch, there's a nap or quiet time, then another period of active playtime, and then, crucially, an hour or so before she begins her bedtime routine, noisy and active play stops and quiet play takes a turn.

This shift from noise, energy, and activity signals to your toddler that it's time to wind down. Put away all the stimulating toys and instead bring out a few books, perhaps a simple puzzle or game (as long as this isn't going to make your toddler frustrated) or some simple drawing items. These quiet, thoughtful activities will keep her occupied until bathtime without fuelling her levels of excitement. Turn off the overhead lights and use lamps around the room to create a softer, more ambient light. Perhaps play some soothing music – avoid pop or children's songs (your toddler might want to sing along), and opt for some classical or gentle music instead.

The return of an absent parent (or parents) during the evening wind down or the subsequent bedtime routine can create a wildly exciting distraction at just the point when your toddler needs calm. Discuss together the options for making sure that she gets to enjoy the company of a returning parent without that being a frantic reunion. See page 49 for some ideas on how to make this work for everyone.

Avoiding bedtime struggles

Winding down also means that you need to avoid any struggles or tantrums during the bedtime routine. Between 18 months and three years old, your toddler is discovering her independence and she'll want to exert her will whenever she thinks she can. Unfortunately, this often means tantrums at bedtime.

Many of the strategies in this book, not least a simple, consistent bedtime routine, will help. A feed, a bath or a general clean, brushing teeth, and a bedtime story all signal consistency, order, and a winding down of the day's activites. You can give your little one a sense of control by letting her choose her pyjamas (give an option of only two), or the blanket she wants on her bed that night (again, limit the choice). See also page 63.

Keeping activities low-key in the run-up to bedtime creates a soothing end to the day.

Consider whether the only time your toddler gets your undivided attention is during the bedtime routine. If it is, her delay tactics and then screams and protestations could be her way of making sure you spend more quality time with her. Try to give her plenty of your time reading, playing games, or discovering new things together during the day, without any other distractions. If you have to go to work, consider putting bedtime back by 30 minutes, so that you have some quality time during the wind down, but ahead of the bedtime routine.

If, despite your best efforts, a tantrum hits, don't give it any favour. If necessary, leave the room to let it blow itself out (making sure she's safe), then when it's over, go back in and give your toddler a cuddle and pop her into bed in the usual way. It's virtually impossible to reason with a tantrumming child, so it's better not to try – you'll only get frustrated.

Choosing a bedtime story

Although your toddler's favourite book might be the one with all the animal sounds, or an action adventure involving a favourite character, a bedtime story should be calming and soothing. If possible, choose one book that you always use at bedtime (or have a choice of three books, and let your toddler choose which one she wants). In this way, the bedtime story becomes a strong trigger that it's time to snuggle down for the night.

Select books with a gentle rhyme or a lilting rhythm. Books about bedtime itself are often well constructed to finish with a sleepy, happy ending. Keep your voice soft as you read, and avoid sound effects or using different voices. Keep it all very simple. If you want to make up your own stories, consider the action and the content carefully – make sure the outcomes are always positive and avoid any drama. Ideally, end the story with an image of bedtime and sweet dreams.

Nightmares and night terrors

Toddlerhood is a time of imaginative play, fantastical paintings, and even simple storytelling. Watch your toddler chatter away to her toys and you'll soon see her imagination at work. The downside of all that creativity, coupled with a greater sense of being separate from you and anxiety about all the new things she is learning, is the possibility that she will begin to have nightmares or night terrors. These are a normal part of growing up, and although distressing to witness, are completely harmless to your child.

Comfort and reassurance will soothe away troubled nights.

Comfort objects

Going to bed with a comfort object, whether a blanket, stuffed toy, or muslin, gives your little one a sense of continuity in her changing world and acts as a portable symbol of the love and security you provide. If your toddler is attached to a stuffed toy, make sure it's safe for pulling at and isn't a choking hazard. Introduce the idea that her comforter will look after her at night.

What is a nightmare?

A nightmare is a frightening dream. These often become apparent around the age of three, although some experts believe they can start earlier. They occur during dreaming (Rapid Eye Movement; see p37) sleep and often during the later part of the night, when periods of REM are longest. A tendency to experience them may be inherited from parents. Toddlers will usually wake screaming or crying from nightmares and may remember them in the morning.

Dealing with nightmares

Because anxiety is thought to be the most common cause of nightmares, your toddler may start to have them simply because of all the new and strange things she is dealing with every day. Consider if something specific may have changed in her life. Has she started nursery? Have you moved her into a new room, bed or even house? Is she potty training? Is there a new baby on the way, or a newborn? If there is a specific reason why you think your toddler may be having nightmares, think of ways to develop her confidence in whatever the trigger might be. Perhaps only time will help – in which case, with reassurance from you during the daytime and gentle soothing at night when she wakes from a nightmare, the phase should soon pass.

Nightmares need soothing when they occur, but try to resist the temptation to bring your child into your bed (unless doing so is acceptable for you and your partner in the long term). Instead, settle her back to sleep with a favourite toy (see box, opposite) and reassurance. Consider a nightlight if the darkness is making matters worse.

What is a night terror?

A night terror is a kind of "parasomnia" – an unwanted behaviour that occurs while asleep. The sleeper doesn't wake up during a night terror, but may sit upright, scream, kick, or thrash about. Like a nightmare, a tendency towards night terrors can be inherited. A night terror occurs in the deepest phase of sleep, often early on in the night, when phases of deep sleep are longest. Your toddler is unlikely to recall the episode in the morning.

Dealing with night terrors

Although it's tempting to wake a child from a night terror, it's better to let it work itself through. Your toddler is in deep sleep, so will be startled and disorientated, and possibly violent, if you wake her while the terror is happening. Instead, make sure she can't fall out of bed or hurt herself, and stay by her side throughout without touching her. When it's over and she appears to be sleeping calmly, gently stroke her cheek and try to bring her to the edge of wakefulness. In this way, she will begin a new sleep cycle, so won't go straight into another phase of deep sleep, and possibly another terror.

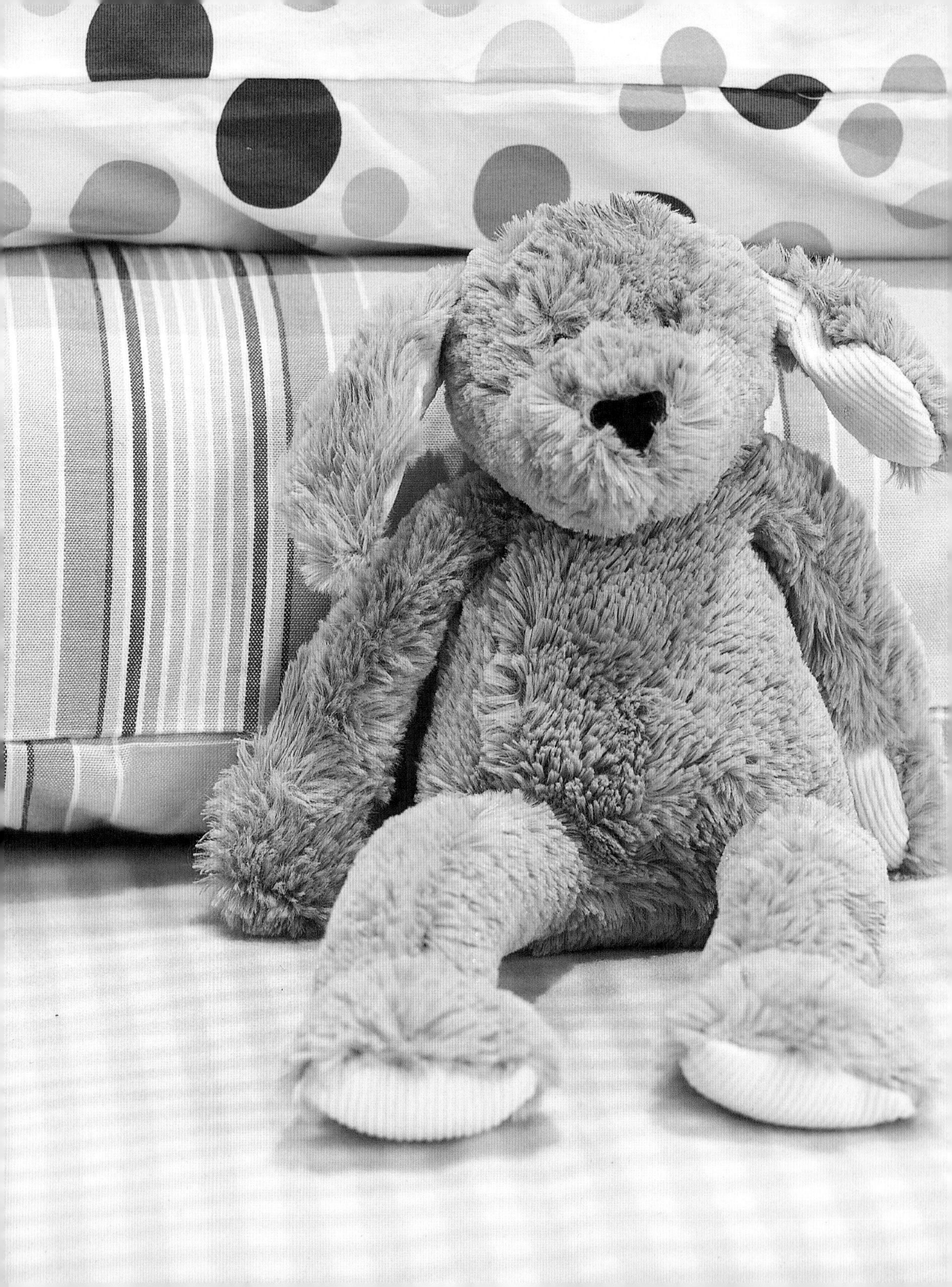

7

Troubleshooting

You think you've done everything you can to make sure that your baby falls asleep easily and sleeps through the night. You've established a good bedtime routine, an active day, a safe sleeping space – and yet still none of you is getting the sleep you need. For decades, sleep and baby experts have devised systems to help parents turn their babies into good sleepers. In this chapter you'll find an overview of all the major strategies for helping your baby to become a confident, healthy nighttime sleeper. Whatever your sleeping issue, choose an approach that best suits your baby, your family, and your lifestyle. Remember that every situation is different and what works for one baby may be far less effective for another. Keep an open mind, persevere, and don't lose heart.

Before you start

If, after months of trying to teach your baby to self-settle, it's still a struggle, it's worth first reviewing your basic sleep practices before implementing a new approach. Once the basics are in place, decide on a technique to suit you all. The approaches in this chapter represent the views of a range of experts – one may provide your solution.

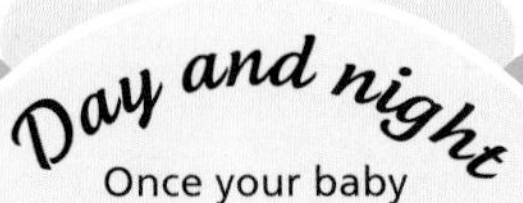

Once your baby was past the newborn phase, at around six to eight weeks old, he was able to start appreciating the difference between day and night. As he grows, continue to emphasize this by keeping the day full of activity and sticking to your wind-down routine as bedtime approaches.

Getting the basics right

The essence of a lifetime of good sleep begins with what experts call good "sleep hygiene", discussed throughout the book, which is about making sure that your baby's sleeping environment, pre-sleep practices, and general lifestyle are all conducive to getting a good night's sleep. If you've got entrenched in bad habits, it can be worth taking a step back to make sure these elements are in place before adopting a sleep-training technique or approach to help (see pp84–93). For some, even with all the basics in place, this may not be enough to settle things: perhaps your baby has a restless temperament, or you've moved house, or have a newborn; or perhaps after many months of bad sleep, you simply want to try a more rigorous approach. However, it's still worth ensuring that these good practices are in place before you embark on a sleep-training method, as this will maximize the likelihood that your baby will respond quickly to whichever technique you choose. Here's a reminder of the basic principles for sleep.

Sleep environment essentials

There are four main aspects to your baby's sleeping environment that it's essential to optimize if you are to give him (and yourself) the best chance of a good night's sleep.

Light. Ensuring that your baby's sleeping environment is dark at nighttime (and flooded with light in the morning) is the most effective way to set his body clock. Put up curtains in his room and use blackout blinds or lining, if necessary. Avoid nightlights or leaving on a landing light if you can. If this is difficult, use a low-wattage bulb. Interestingly, the brain doesn't register red light as dawn light, so a low-wattage red bulb is best (see p31).

In the morning, open the curtains or draw up the blinds to let the sunlight flood in. This

tells your baby's body clock that it's morning.
Noise. Although some babies will sleep better with "white noise", such as the hum of a fan, in the background, in general try to make the nighttime sleeping environment as quiet as possible. This is another marker for your baby that there's a different mood for sleep. Most babies will sleep through a regular noise, such as the constant hum of traffic, but loud noises can startle them. If you live on a street that has intermittent traffic, or a dog that barks, heavy curtains will help to muffle the sound. Double or secondary glazing, though, is ideal.
Temperature. Your baby's sleeping space should be neither too hot nor too cold, but if in doubt, err on the slightly cool side and add a blanket if needed. Sleep experts suggest a temperature of between 16 and 20°C (60.8 and 68°F), with 18°C (64.4°F) as ideal. Use a cotton

The right bedtime conditions set your child up for a sound night's sleep.

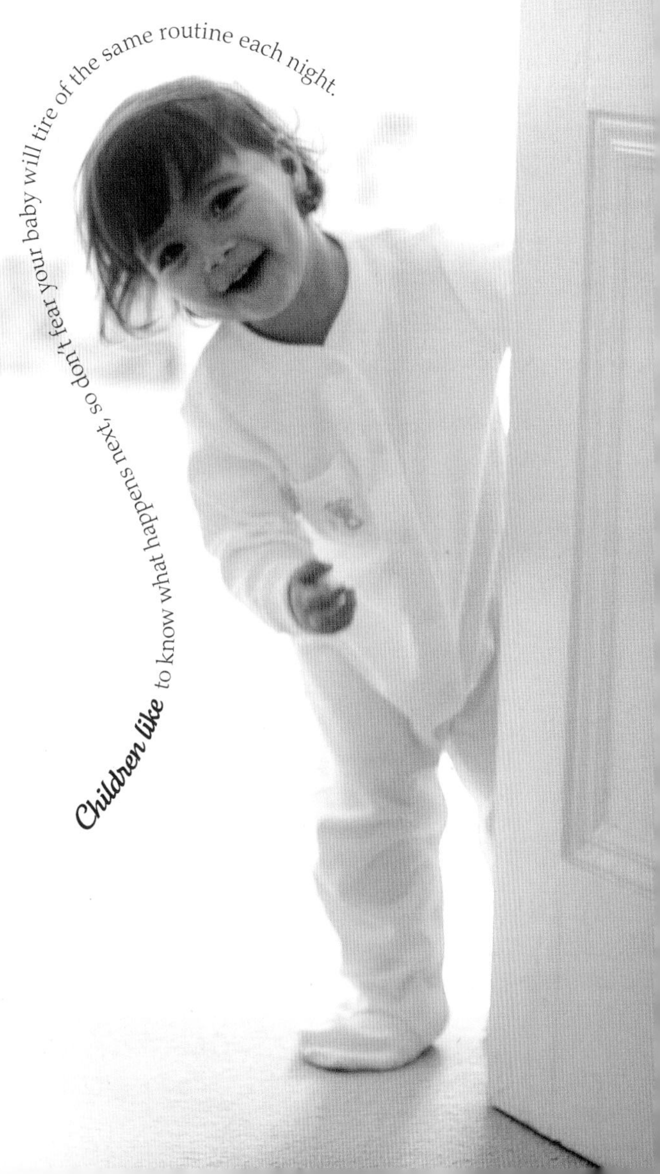

sheet above and below him and put him in cotton sleepwear. Cotton wicks away sweat if he gets slightly warm, keeping his body temperature constant, but also keeps him warm if he's cool. If he wakes around three or four in the morning, consider whether he might be too cold – this is when body temperature is at its lowest. He'll find it hard to fall asleep if his room is too warm, because his body temperature needs to be falling to trigger the mechanisms of sleep.
Sleeping place. Whether your baby sleeps in a cot or a crib, or in your bed, ensure there's nothing that he could get tangled up in. Use cotton bedding (see above) and layers of blankets rather than a duvet. Make sure that his mattress supports him, is level, and that, if he's in a cot or crib, he can't catch his fingers in any parts, or wedge himself between the mattress and the structure of the cot.

Children like to know what happens next, so don't fear your baby will tire of the same routine each night.

Co-sleeping

Sharing a bed together is one of the most nurturing and natural ways to bond with your baby. It has been in practice since the beginning of time, and is still commonplace in cultures all over the world. As with any sleep method, though, co-sleeping is not without its potential problems. If co-sleeping is the course you decide upon, how can you make it work for you all?

The benefits of co-sleeping

In the first few months of life, your baby thinks he is still a part of you. Co-sleeping advocates claim that very young babies can be anxious when in a separate sleeping place, and believe the most natural, secure place for your baby to sleep is next to you, listening to your breathing.

If he wakes frequently at night, or finds it hard to fall asleep, co-sleeping can help your baby feel secure so that he learns to drift off easily, and fall back to sleep easily when he wakes. Furthermore, if you're breastfeeding, you will be able to latch him on at his first murmurs, and you can doze while he feeds. Some experts suggest that you can synchronize your sleep cycles with those of your baby, with the overall benefit that everyone's sleep is improved. Also, if you are at work all day (or your partner is), co-sleeping can be a wonderful way to strengthen your bonds with your baby.

Co-sleeping problems

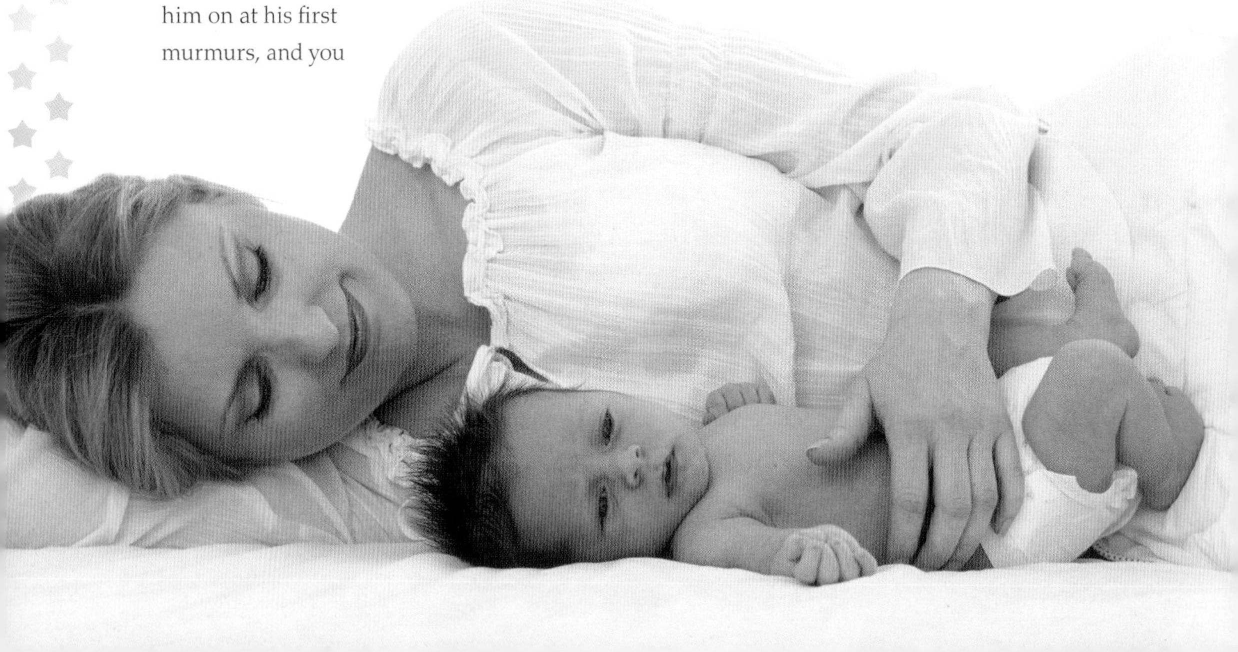

Although it seems perfectly natural to sleep with your baby near you, doing so is not without its problems. Some parents find their baby's murmuring and fidgeting results in a fitful night for all. Equally, your baby might sleep less soundly as a result of your noises and movements. Or you may worry about rolling on to your baby, which may affect your ability to sleep deeply. See pages 22–3 for co-sleeping safety guidelines. Some parents want to continue co-sleeping with their toddler, but find this is more difficult as their baby grows. If you don't want to make the break to separate sleeping spaces just yet, or need strategies to deal with elements of co-sleeping, consider some of the practical ideas below.

Working together

Whether or not to co-sleep is a decision that you and your partner must come to together. Consider the effects on your relationship with each other. With your baby in your bed, there may be fewer opportunities for intimacy, so you both need to be happy with this arrangement for it to work.

Making it work

There are two main ways to co-sleep. The first is to have your baby in your own bed, and the second is to have a cot with a removable side that you position up against your bed (which has the benefit of giving your baby his own space if any of you needs it). Whichever method you choose, there are practical ways to make this sleeping arrangement work for all of you.

For many, co-sleeping can be a wholly positive experience for the family.

• If you are sleeping all together in one bed, there are clear benefits to having a king-size bed, if possible. You will each have plenty of space, and co-sleeping will continue to be a comfortable option as your baby grows.

• A bed "nest" for your baby can work well if you are disturbed by your baby's movements, or he is disturbed by yours. This is a portable infant bed, suitable for babies up to four months, that you place in between you and your partner. Your baby has his own divided space next to you so there is no danger of you rolling on top of him.

• Try a meshed guard-rail suitable for a young baby on one side of the bed. After a feed, settle your baby between mum and the rail – mothers are thought to be more instinctively aware of where their baby is. This also allows you to maintain intimacy with your partner.

• Putting your mattress on the floor removes the worry about your baby falling out of bed. Ideally place the mattress up against the wall.

If you have an open-sided cot next to your bed, make sure the levels of your mattress and the baby's mattress are exactly the same and that your baby could not become wedged between the two beds. If your baby is sleeping in your bed and you need to get out of bed at night, or wake earlier than your baby in the morning, you will need to move him to a crib, cot, or Moses basket as he should never be left unattended in your bed.

No cry

The no-cry method focuses on your baby's inherent need for closeness and reassurance, and is in tune with the fact that babies – at least in their first few months of life – don't cry to manipulate you.

The technique

Techniques vary, but broadly the no-cry method involves nursing your baby, then putting him down when he's on the cusp of sleep. While some methods suggest waiting until your baby is fully asleep, most sleep experts agree that it's better for a baby to learn to fall asleep without associating doing so with sucking on a bottle or nursing.

Once he's almost asleep, put him in his sleeping place. If he cries, pick him up to reassure him, and when he's calm again, put him down. The idea is that he is not left to cry; rather, he's reassured by your response, and so develops the confidence to fall asleep easily. You can also use a word or phrase to indicate it's sleep time, such as "Shhh" or "It's sleep time now." Repeat this as you rock, stroke, and reassure him to sleep (or back to sleep). Eventually, the phrase alone is enough to induce sleep.

During the night, as soon as he murmurs for a feed, you give it. For this reason, many no-cry methods encourage co-sleeping (see pp84–5), at least in the early months.

Some parents want their little one to be sure of their constant, quick response.

Is this technique for you?

The system is best suited to younger babies, although has been used and is said to work for babies all the way into toddlerhood. It's considered one of the most gentle ways to encourage your child to sleep as at no point does he become anxious that you are not there. Advocates claim that not only does he learn to sleep through the night, but he is less likely to develop traumatic associations about sleep, and more likely to grow up to be a confident and secure individual. The downside of the method is that it can take a long time to have a self-settler – it may be weeks or even months before your baby is able to soothe himself to sleep and sleep through the night.

Pick up–put down

This technique varies according to the age of your baby, but the aim is to teach him that you are always there so that he trusts in sleep and develops no sense of abandonment.

Newborn technique

Until your baby is three or four months old, pick up–put down is known as "shush–pat". Choose a key phrase (like "shhh") that you say when you put him in his crib. If he cries, go to him and pat him – on his tummy or arm – while repeating the phrase (some babies may need only a pat). If he doesn't settle in a few minutes, pick him up and keep patting him and repeating the phrase. As soon as he calms, put him back in his crib. Pat him and repeat the phrase once more, then move away from him, out of sight if you can. Repeat as often as needed until he falls asleep.

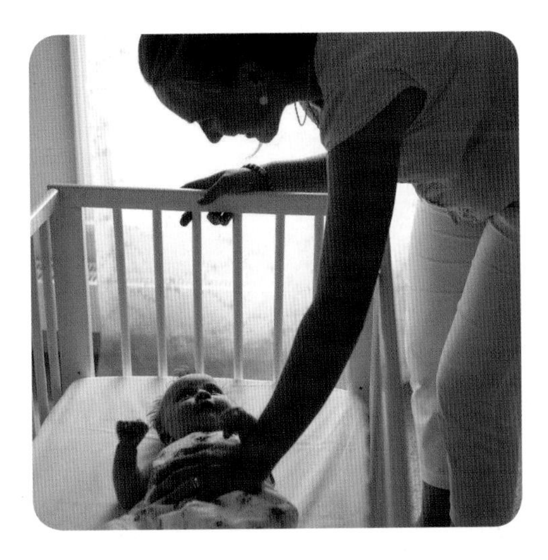

From four months

If you've been doing shush–pat from birth and it isn't quite working, or you're just starting, from four months old it becomes "pick up–put down". When he cries, try shush–pat, but if that doesn't work, pick him up. Once he settles, or if you've been holding him for five minutes, put him down, repeating your phrase. If he doesn't settle, repeat the process until he falls asleep.

At six months old, babies may struggle as you try to pick them up. The safest thing to do is to put him down straight away and let him thrash it out. Keep your hand gently on his tummy so that he knows you're there, then when he's calm repeat your key phrase and move away, as before. Babies around eight months old are best settled using shush–pat again, as they are more likely to wake fully and be more disturbed if you pick them up from their bed.

Is this technique for you?

The pick up–put down technique is a gentle way to teach your baby to settle. You're with him the whole time he is crying, so he develops trust and self-confidence and never feels abandoned. However, the method does require patience and resilience (one settling session can take anything from 10 minutes to hours). While some parents find success within days, others can find it takes a month or more to break the cycle of crying.

Gradual withdrawal

Babies will fall asleep when they feel most secure, which means that many quickly grow used to falling asleep in your arms during the first weeks and months of life. The gradual withdrawal method is the technique most suited to teaching a clingy baby to self-settle.

The technique

Gradual withdrawal is just as the name suggests. Very slowly, over several nights, or weeks, and in increments barely perceptible to your baby, you withdraw your physical presence as he falls asleep, until at last he falls asleep without you.

How it works

If your baby is used to falling asleep in your arms, or with you patting or stroking him, the technique might involve gradually making strokes or pats lighter until your hand skims the cotton of his bedclothes. You can have a key phrase, too, such as "Shhh" or "Time for sleep", which, once you have withdrawn your touch, is enough to trigger sleep in itself.

If he has been used to you lying next to him as he falls asleep, or wants you in the room with him, he needs the confidence to settle even if you're out of sight.

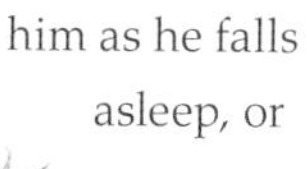

On the first night, put a chair next to his cot (or bed if he's a toddler) where you sit while he falls asleep. Repeat your sleep phrase quietly until he falls asleep, then wait for five minutes before leaving the room. Once he's used to this, move your chair a short distance from the cot, using your sleep phrase as before. Each night, move the chair a little further away until you are just outside the door. Eventually he will learn to settle himself as soon as you say your sleep phrase and leave the room.

This gentle method to help a clingy baby to settle works for many families.

Is this technique for you?

Gradual withdrawal maintains your baby's trust in your presence, but at the same time gives him the confidence to put himself to sleep. It will usually take only around 14 days to get your baby to self-settle in this way, but for some it can take up to four weeks. As with all the techniques, you will need to be patient and consistent to see results.

Rapid return

Once your baby is in a bed, has found his feet, and can get in and out of his bed and room, the problem of getting him to go to sleep is exacerbated by his newfound freedom. Rapid return may provide a solution.

The technique

In general, children will give up a certain behaviour if they think something boring or unwanted happens as a result. Rapid return capitalizes on this low tolerance.

Getting out of bed straight away

If your toddler follows you out of his room at bedtime, take him by the hand and gently, but firmly, and with as little eye contact as possible, put him back in his bed. Repeat your goodnight phrase, if you have one, and leave the room. Don't chastise him – simply put him back in bed. If he gets out again, do exactly the same thing. If he protests or drags his feet, pick him up if necessary, but make no eye contact, and put him back as matter-of-factly as possible.

Once he is finally in his bed and staying there, leave him to try to settle himself, but if he continues to cry, go in and use your usual bedtime sound or phrase to reassure him and then leave the room again. Keep going back at increasing intervals until he falls asleep.

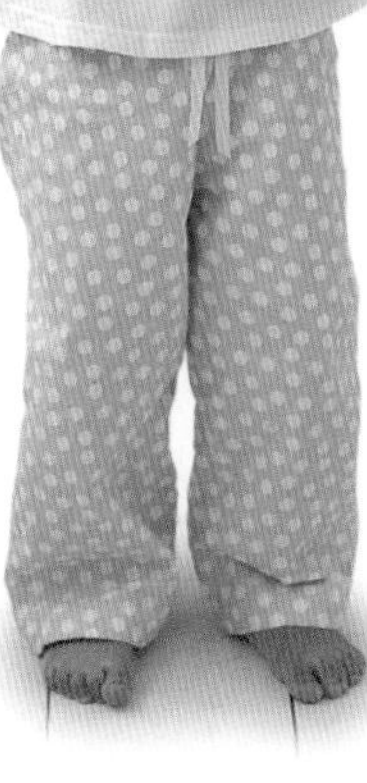

Middle-of-the-night visiting

It's not unusual for toddlers to wake up fully between sleep cycles in the night. Whereas once he might have called out for you to go to him, he now has the freedom to find you.

Don't encourage him in to your bed. Instead, get up yourself and, without telling him off, take him by the hand back to his bed. Make this as monotonous a process as possible, and repeat for as often as he comes back to your room. If he cries when you put him back into bed, soothe him with a gentle pat and your goodnight sound or phrase. Then, when he's calm, leave the room.

Eventually, when your toddler realizes that the results of his nighttime adventures are really very boring, he should give up getting out of bed at all.

Is this technique for you?

Because it involves you getting up and returning your toddler to bed every time he gets out, the process can be hard to stick to and can require strength of will before you see results. Some toddlers may give up and stay in bed in a matter of days or a week; for others, you may find yourself going back and forth between rooms for more than a month.

Controlled crying

All babies cry. In fact, at the beginning of their lives it is their only effective means of communication, and they will use different types of cry to convey different needs (see p41). Nonetheless, all babies need to learn to settle themselves to sleep, and controlled crying, best done after six months, can be a way to teach your baby that bedtime in itself is not a reason to cry.

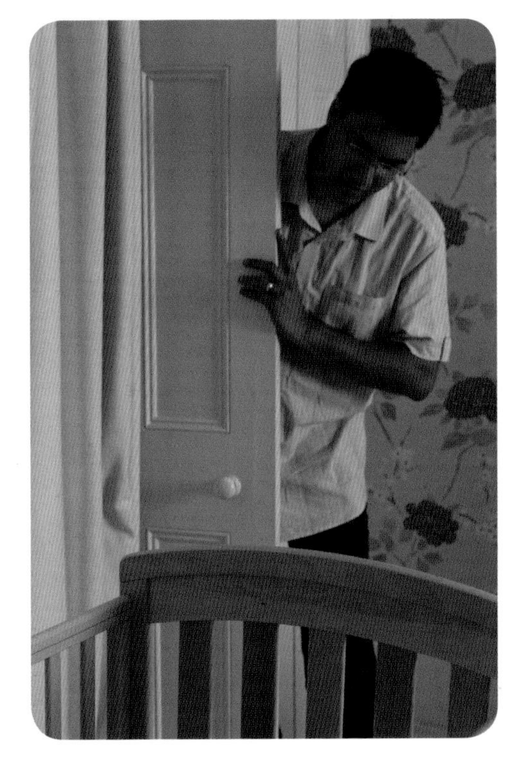

Choosing this technique takes resolve, and confidence that it's right for your baby.

The technique

Follow your bedtime routine in the usual way, then put your baby in his cot. If he begins to cry, say your goodnight, but don't touch him, then leave the room. Leave him to cry for a minute or so (but no longer than five minutes; agree with your partner what the starting point is going to be, so that you are both doing the same thing), and if he is still crying, go back into the room and reassure him with only a phrase or comment, such as "There's no need to cry. Mummy and Daddy are here." Then leave the room. If the crying continues, increase the amount of time you leave it before you return and repeat the phrase. The amount of time you add is up to you, and your resolve. Some parents can manage only minute-long increments (going in after one minute, then two minutes, then three minutes, and so on), while others add five minutes at a time (going in after five minutes, then 10 minutes, and so on) or longer. It doesn't really matter what you go for, as long as you are consistent.

Once his cries turn into more of a whimper, try to avoid going back in at all – this could be a sign that he is settling himself to sleep. If, however, he starts to cry loudly again, continue the process. Most sleep experts agree that it will take around an hour or so for a baby finally to fall asleep soundly.

Why wait?

Experts advise waiting until your baby is six months old before trying controlled crying. This is because by then you have an established bond and he has some sense of himself and his control over his world. He's also reaching a stage where he can consciously use crying as a means of communication.

Waking in the night

If your baby starts to cry for you in the night, leave him to cry for the amount of time you and your partner have agreed, and then start the process from the beginning, going in at increasing intervals.

Is this technique for you?

Some experts oppose controlled crying, claiming that this sleep-training technique hampers social development, making it harder for a baby to build trust, and that it can cause unnecessary stress. However, advocates of this method of settling babies claim that controlled crying is no more harmful to a baby than more nurturing sleep-training techniques and practices.

Supporters of controlled crying believe that the process of learning to self-settle is quicker for your baby because he doesn't learn that crying gets him positive attention in the form of your touch or extended presence. They claim that more gentle methods teach babies that crying brings positive attention, such as cuddles and strokes, and so it takes your baby longer to get the message that it is time to sleep rather than interact.

You will need to have firm resolve to make this technique work – it can be distressing to hear your baby crying for extended periods of time and it goes against all instinct to ignore him. Use a watch to time your intervals precisely and take it in turns with your partner to go in. This will relieve the pressure on either one of you. It will also teach your baby that different people may settle him.

Once you begin the technique, and if you apply it consistently, you will almost certainly see positive effects within a few days to a week. As always, some babies take longer, and most have a setback at some time or another.

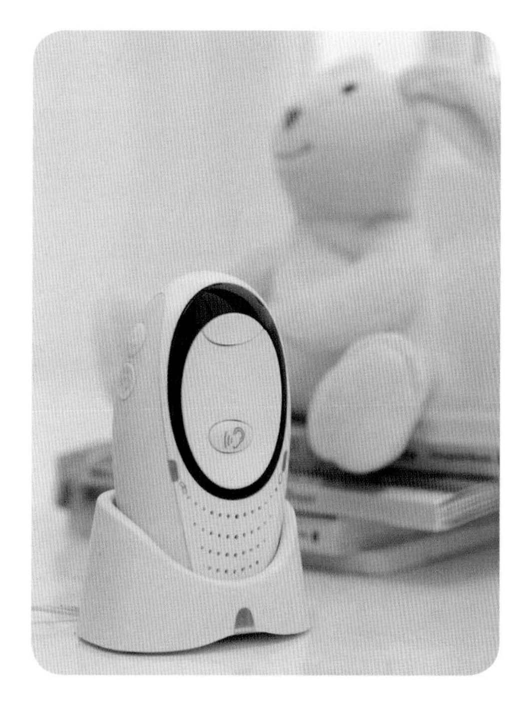

Crying it out

In clinical terms, crying it out is a form of "extinction", a psychologist's word meaning to withhold a response to change behaviour. In the case of crying it out, the parent withholds attention, and in doing so teaches their baby that crying doesn't bring him rewards, so he stops doing it.

The technique

The terms "crying it out" and "controlled crying" (see pp90–1) are sometimes used interchangeably. However, in the strictest sense, crying it out is a more extreme form of controlled crying in which you ignore your baby's cries until he gives up and goes to sleep.

If you wish to try this technique, follow your bedtime routine, then put your baby to bed as usual, leaving the room with the reassurances you usually give. If he subsequently calls out for you, you ignore his cries as well as any subsequent protestations he makes.

Is this technique for you?

Ignoring a crying baby requires huge amounts of willpower and resolve and can be incredibly difficult for parents. Some experts suggest that, as with controlled crying, leaving your baby to cry could cause detrimental changes in the developing brain. However, while the possible risks are similar to controlled crying, results are often fast, and you could have your baby sleeping through the night in just two or three days. Advocates of this method argue that it is ultimately kinder than a more long-winded process. Don't underestimate, though, how long every minute of your baby's cries will seem to you. Make sure both you and your partner are on board with the technique so you can support each other. If you prefer, you might want to agree on an upper time limit, of say 15 minutes, for leaving your baby to cry. Don't attempt this method until your baby is at least seven months old so that he has already learned to trust you.

Leaving your baby to cry can be distressing for you as well as for your baby.

Finally, some safety notices. You won't be returning to the room, so make sure your baby can't come to any harm (see pp34–5 on cot safety). If you can, put a mirror or visual baby monitor in his room so that you can at least see if he seems to be in a lot of distress. Bear in mind, too, that some babies can scream so much that they make themselves sick, or even hyperventilate. Some in deep distress may breath-hold, forcing themselves to pass out.

If you think that you and your partner would find this technique too harsh, but are looking for a quicker solution than the more nurturing settling methods would give, you could consider using controlled crying (see pp90–1) instead.

Praise and reward

Once your baby gets to toddlerhood, he will fully understand the notions of praise and reward and he will love it when he does something right and is greeted with huge smiles, stars, and perhaps even a well-earned treat. Capitalizing on the idea of "positive parenting", this technique is less about ignoring unwanted behaviour and all about celebrating good behaviour.

The technique

First, decide what behaviour to reward. Keep goals simple so that your toddler can recognize and understand them. A chart with pictures to represent the aims is a good idea (you can cut pictures from magazines if you aren't artistic – involve your toddler in making the chart, too). For example, if he keeps getting out of bed, he could get a sticker for staying in bed all night. You could also reward elements of the bedtime routine: good tooth brushing, kissing his teddies, saying goodnight nicely. If some goals are easily achievable, he will feel motivated to focus on the more challenging ones, too.

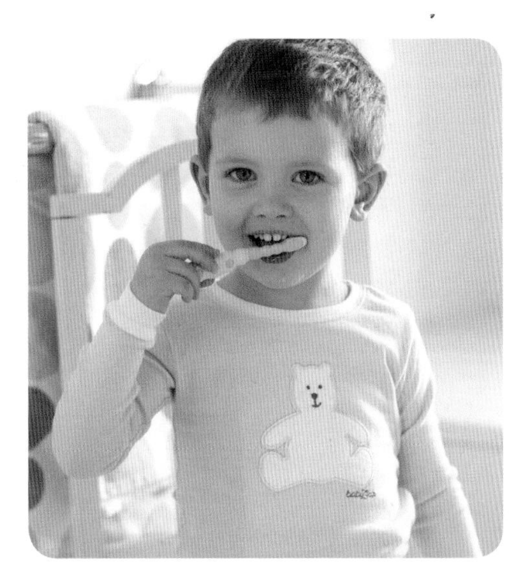

You could also have a system of "strikes". You might, for example, give "three strikes" before your toddler loses his opportunity for stickers: three chances at staying in bed when he's told. If he gets up a fourth time, he doesn't get his sticker for that night.

Give out stickers in the morning. Praise him and decide on a treat at the end of the week if he reaches his target. Make sure that both you and your partner are clear on what stickers are for and on the treat – if you reward different behaviours, your toddler will get confused. And, if collecting stickers is the way to earn a treat, don't forget to give the treat! Your toddler has earned it and will lose interest if he doesn't see the fruits of his labours.

Is this technique for you?

This works for toddlers and preschoolers who are motivated by the desire to please. Some children are just not interested in sticker charts.

Use the reward system only if your goals are simple and clear, such as staying in bed all night or not getting up in the morning before a certain time. Poorly defined goals are hard for your toddler to understand and for you to reward consistently.

Index

Acknowledgments

Authors's acknowledgments

My sincere and heartfelt thanks to Peggy Vance and Anna Davidson at Dorling Kindersley for asking me to write the book – and to Claire Cross for her impeccable guidance, thoughtfulness and reassurance throughout the process. Thank you, too, to Chris Idzikowski, who first lured me into the fascinating subject of the science of sleep. Most of all, though, love and thanks to Eliza and Martha, my beautiful larks, whose practical instruction has proved invaluable (!), and to Simon – for being so much better at lack of sleep than me and for everything else that matters.

Publisher's acknowledgments

Dorling Kindersley would like to thank Claire Wedderburn-Maxwell for proofreading, and Michèle Clarke for the index.

Resources

www.cry-sis.org.uk
Support for parents with crying, sleepless, and restless babies

www.lullabytrust.org.uk
Information on safe sleeping for babies

www.nhs.uk
Information on parenting and babycare

www.gingerbread.org.uk
Advice and practical support for single parents

www.familylives.org.uk
Parenting and family support with chat forum. National helpline 0808 800 2222

www.babycentre.co.uk
Online resource for new and expectant parents with chat forum

www.mumsnet.com
Online forum for parents run by parents. Information and discussion threads on all aspects of parenting

www.forums.parentingclub.com
Online forum with support and tips

www.tamba.org.uk
The Twins and Multiple Birth Association. Advice and support on raising twins

www.breastfeedingnetwork.org.uk
Support and information for breastfeeding women. National helpline 0300 100 0212

www.abm.me.uk
Association of Breastfeeding Mothers – offers support and advice